FAR FROM HELP!
Backcountry Medical Care

Peter Steele's lifelong love of wilderness and mountains began with Outward Bound and quickly grew to include climbs in Britain, the Pyrenees, the Alps, and a crossing of the Sahara by camel to explore and photograph the extinct villages of Tibesti. After receiving his degree in medicine in 1960, he drove overland to Nepal with wife Sarah, a nurse, where they worked in a Kathmandu hospital and explored the western end of the Dhaulagiri range. He ran the Grenfell Flying Doctor service in Northern Labrador in 1964 before returning to Bristol, England to resume his frequently interrupted surgical career. Peter and Sarah next crossed the Bhutan Himalayas, with their two children under four years old, an adventure charmingly told in *Two and Two Halves to Bhutan*. He was a climbing medical officer for the 1971 International Everest Expedition; he described the tragedy and controversy in *Doctor on Everest*.

Peter hitch-hiked around South America with his ten-year-old son before moving to the Yukon in 1975 to practice family medicine. He has since climbed, skied, and canoed throughout the Yukon wilderness, and has made two long overland journeys with Sarah; through China, Tibet and India in 1986 and from Nairobi, Kenya to Capetown in 1989. He says he is, "still searching for nirvana but has yet to find anything closer to it than the Yukon."

Far From Help! is based on the author's wide experience of providing medical care in some of the world's more remote places.

FAR FROM HELP!
Backcountry Medical Care

by Peter Steele

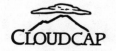

CLOUDCAP

Published in North America by:
CLOUDCAP, Box 27344, Seattle, WA 98125

ISBN 0-938567-19-5 (cloth)
     0-938567-26-8 (paper)

[Some of the material in this edition previously appeared in
Medical Care for Mountaineers, published in 1976 by Heinemann,
London; and *Medical Handbook for Mountaineers*, published in
1988 by Constable, London]

Manufactured in the United States of America

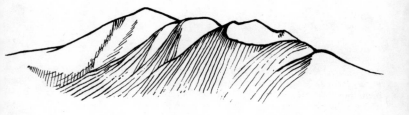

To Lucy

Contents

List of Diagrams

(Drawings by Jean McAllister)

Acknowledgements

Monty Alford, mountaineer; Steve Bezruchka, Everest doctor; Dave Boon, ENT surgeon; Frank Buffam, opthalmologist; Jeremy Carless, family physician; Charles Clarke, Everest doctor; Peter Cummings, emergency physician; Peter Currie, anesthetist; Baman Daver, plastic surgeon; Jim Dalrymple, general surgeon; John Dickinson, physician in Nepal; Andrew Elkington, opthalmologist; Jon Elliott, physician; Max Fleming, father-in-law; John Hayward, cold physiologist; Tony Holmyard, outdoor educator; Charles Houston, altitude physician; Judy Isaac-Renton, tropical medicine; John James, family physician; Eric Langmuir, mountaineer; Peter Lord, general surgeon; Hector Mackenzie, wilderness guide; Paul Millac, neurologist; Wayne Merry, mountaineer; Bruce Paton, vascular surgeon; Ron Pearson, dental surgeon; Drummond Rennie, altitude physician; Gil Roberts, Everest Doctor; Barney Rosedale, Everest Doctor; Sandy Sanders, clinical pharmacologist; Chris Shank, mountaineer; Ann Skidmore, microbiologist; Ian Taylor, plastic surgeon; Frank Timmermans, general surgeon; Michael Ward, Everest surgeon; Andy Williams, high altitude pilot.

Preface

In this book my aim is to help active outdoorsmen in the wilderness to muster their wits in order to keep alive the victim of an accident or a medical emergency during the first few shattering minutes, and to prevent any worsening before skilled care is reached.

A recurring question of helpful critics has been, "who is your audience?" The book is for anyone who ventures into the wilderness — a teacher leading school children on a hike, a maestro mountaineer on some alpine north face, or a young doctor trekking with a party in the Himalaya. Medical knowledge will vary widely, yet I have written one book in hope of interesting everyone — a dangerous task.

In order to separate information that should be universal from more technical detail, different print sizes are used. This allows matters of interest to the more medically trained reader, or those superfluous to immediate practical help, to be retained in small print:

Without burdening the average person with gobblegook.

I struggled with the question of how to refer to the injured party — victim, casualty, patient, trekker, person — and settled on victim, who I also generally refer to as male solely for ease of syntax. I ask indulgence of female readers.

*Economy of words, clear meaning and plain English are my foremost aim **throughout**.* I try to avoid medical jargon, the cloak of mystique under which many doctors hide. Occasionally a medical word is apt; then I am not shy to use it.

Many friends, experts in their own fields, have been generous with their criticism; my debt to them is immense. They have sealed the book with authority and helped me to make it as accurate, yet understandable, as possible. Any errors or omissions are my responsibility, but I would much appreciate hearing about them.

Introduction

Accidents and medical crises create anxiety and tension. Even experienced emergency physicians feel adrenalin coursing through their veins when an ambulance siren wails and strobe lights flash, as they wonder what horror will unfold when the ambulance doors open. In wilderness you may be *far from help* with few resources and with meager medical knowledge, a situation that will readily cause panic and confusion unless you, the rescuer, keep a cool head and act decisively.

Assess the the victim's condition and decide what needs doing immediately in order to prevent him worsening or dying before you can get help. During this lonely, anxious time, the sight of blood and a cadaverous victim may lead you to flounder unless you marshal your thoughts clearly and quickly.

Accident Prevention

Prevention, if properly applied, would make this book redundant. In an imperfect world prevention, sadly, will never be totally effective. Wilderness is hazardous, and some people will get hurt, and may die, whatever precautions are taken. Prevention demands learning new skills in order to reduce the dangers inherent in the outdoors. Learn everything possible about wilderness before venturing into it, apply common sense while there, and judge when to accept defeat and to turn back rather than press on towards disaster. Only a thorough apprenticeship will prepare you to handle these dangers, which can be reduced by honing your technical skills in order to become a well-rounded outdoorsman. Medical problems of wilderness are often problems of wilderness more than of medicine. It is comparatively easy to splint a broken leg and treat the pain, but how to evacuate the victim safely without suffering from further injury, illness, or hypothermia will depend on hard-won skill and experience.

A big medical kit and all the newest gear will not lessen the dangers. Carry only essentials because, if weighed down by impedimenta, energy needed for coping with the unexpected will be expended fruitlessly.

Emergency doctors can do little outside hospital. A well-trained first-aider may be more useful in wilderness than a doctor who is ignorant of the special problems of remote places. An MD (or whatever) after his name does not necessarily mean he is any better than a competent outdoorsman who has learned the basic medical skills. Illnesses are as often cured by Nature as by the doctor.

The Law

Good Samaritans in the outdoors are unlikely to fall foul of the law when their attempts to save life fail provided they apply conscientiously skills learned, and stick within their capabilities. Legal action looms large these days, so the lily-livered should stay well away from the medical care business. Rescuing, like adventure, carries risks but we still attempt both.

1 THE ACCIDENT SCENE

After an accident one person should take charge in order to prevent confusion from too many people offering smart ideas. If reticent to lead, give your support to a leader who has first-aid experience, and thereby influence the operation from a back seat.

Plan a safe approach to the victim. In mountains, for example, come from below or from the side, but not from above where a rock-slide or an avalanche may start. Move the victim to safe level ground, if possible, make a shelter, and keep him warm. Undo tight clothing and equipment, cutting along seams if necessary. Do the minimum first-aid on site in order to stabilize him until skilled medical help, which may yet be far away, is reached. Panicking bystanders put pressure on a first-aider to DO something, but knowing what NOT TO DO is more important. Action for action's sake, may lead to meddlesome interference. Whatever you may do, not-so-bad accident victims tend to get better, while very bad ones tend to get worse and die.

Care of the victim

Care means total care of the whole person — frightened, anxious, and in pain — not just bandaging his wounds. First, reassure and comfort him, especially if it seems he may die. Compassion needs no medical skill, just warm caring humanity. Call him by name; tell him your name, who you are, and your first-aid qualifications in order to bolster his confidence. Touching helps to establish a bond of trust; hold his hand or lay your hand on his shoulder.

Make him as comfortable as the ground will allow; let him pee if he needs to. While waiting for, and during, the rescue, insulation from the cold ground below is just as important as piling clothes on top to keep him warm. An immobile, injured person can quickly suffer hypothermia, which may be more lethal than his injury.

Moving him may cause pain so give warning to avoid surprise. Withold pain-killers usually until after examining him in order not to disguise pain and obscure physical signs; but if pain is severe, treat it regardless. Examine him carefully and thoroughly, thereby reassuring him your care will be thorough, but also lessening the chance of missing some important sign.

Assess the victim and then explain carefully his situation, telling no lies. He will be anxious about being crippled, that his job will be jeopardized, what his family will say. Inevitably he will feel guilty at being the cause of so much trouble; even if the accident was his fault, blaming him is pointless. From now on he will be totally dependent on your rescue skills and such dependence erodes self-esteem. Encourage him to discuss the accident in order to dispel guilt and embarrassment.

Make a plan of action, discuss it with the victim, and try to involve him in his own rescue. He may be able to hold a rope, or light a stove to boil water for tea while you attend to other things.

Assessment

A quick but careful scrutiny of the victim should reveal the main injuries or problems; a full and leisurely exam can follow once this most urgent question has been answered:

Is the victim in immediate danger of dying?

In wilderness, as in the city, life is in imminent danger in cases of airway block, chest injury, severe head injury, or massive bleeding. In any of these conditions, provided not patently hopeless, act before trying to identify the precise cause of trouble. In other cases there is usually sufficient time to ask the victim what happened, and to examine him thoroughly in order to assemble the facts before reaching a reasoned diagnosis. Doctors and medical personnel are trained this way and other people should do the same. Some of the terms used in the following paragraphs of this section may be unclear unless the relevant chapters in the book have been read.

The injured person is most likely to die from:

  —extensive damage to the entire body caused by the accident
  —inability to breathe owing to airway block or chest injury
  —severe head injury and the sequels of unconsciousness
  —profuse bleeding causing shock and heart stop

Airway — listen for the snoring breathing of airway block. Turn the victim into the draining position, tilt the head, remove secretions, lift the jaw and insert an oral airway. Do not make a pillow for his head.

Breathing — listen for croaking stridor; look for the rise and fall of the lower chest and upper abdomen — if absent start rescue breathing.

Circulation — look for blood from an exposed wound; feel under the victim for pooled blood soaked in clothing and lying unnoticed behind the back or head. Control bleeding with steady pressure directly on the wound. In order to assess the circulation feel the pulse at the wrist or neck, and notice the speed of return of color to the nail bed after blanching with pressure. Look at the face for the pallor of shock and the blue color of cyanosis.

Neurological — first and most important, assess the conscious level according to the Glasgow Coma Scale. Then look at the pupils for difference in size indicating bleeding inside the skull, and at the nose and ears for cerebro-spinal fluid leaking from a fracture at the base of the skull.

Bones — feel the skull, chest and pelvis for fractures, and move the limbs gently watching the victim's face for wincing owing to pain. Splint fractures and reduce dislocations if possible.

EXAM
Make sure the victim is not in urgent need of life-saving attention, and if necessary move him to a safe place (out of danger of rockfall or avalanche) and with space to move around, do a thorough and leisurely exam.

The scheme: Exam, Ask, Look, Listen, Feel, Move, Act, Rx (= treat) — is a rough framework for most of the chapters in this book. Plain English words are explicit and preferable to verbose jargon such as examination, observation, auscultation, palpation.

ASK
Ask a conscious person for a full story of the accident or illness

and of any symptoms (the feelings of which he complains); if the victim is unconscious ask a witness. Follow a similar routine every time you ask a story and examine someone; in this way, as in a pilot's pre-flight check, nothing important will be missed. Always write down findings immediately because details may be forgotten later. An accurate written record will assist the receiving hospital doctor. Whatever scheme is adopted stick to it so it becomes routine.

General questions
— name, age, address, next of kin, occupation
— chief complaint; use the person's own words to write a sequential story of the accident or illness, asking especially about pain: time of onset, nature, severity, change in character
— past illnesses and surgery, with dates
— present medication; look for a Medic-Alert bracelet or medallion
— allergies; to drugs, foods, and insect stings.

Systematic history
— heart: chest pain, palpitations, shortness of breath, swelling of ankles
— chest: cough and sputum, difficult breathing, wheeze or croup
— gut: pain, appetite, nausea, vomiting, indigestion, constipation or diarrhea
— urine: frequency, pain, burning, volume and color
— nerves: conscious level; seizures, faints, headaches; loss of power or sensation, numbness or tingling.
— motor: pain or weakness in bones, muscles or joints; abnormal gait and walking.

EXAM
Examine the victim under shelter, with adequate light, and un-dressed so nothing is obscured by clothing; remember the back as well as the front. Cold hands will make him flinch and you will learn nothing. The order in which the victim is examined and the findings recorded is unimportant so long as the scheme is unvarying. Start at the crown of the head and work towards the feet.

When examining a paired part, for example a limb or one side of the chest, always have the opposite side exposed for comparison; slight swelling or deformity becomes obvious when compared with the normal side. Negative findings may be as important as positive ones. Perform every step of the exam even if the injury or illness appears obvious at first sight, because a secondary condition, obscured by an exigent chief complaint, may be equally significant. The victim needs reassessing frequently, at least every half hour, because much can change after the initial exam.

The following outline is a rough check-list; refer to specific chapters for more details. Examining someone requires practice and skill, but all doctors were inept medical students once. This scheme presupposes no specialized medical equipment.

General appearance
— sick or well (an impression formed by instinct rather than by specific signs)
— consciousness and co-operation
— demeanor (lying still, rolling around)
— pain, temperature, fever
— skin color: anemia (pink color of lower inner eyelid or fingernail), cyanosis (blue color inside lips), jaundice (yellow color of whites of the eyes)
— skin eruptions
— hands: tell a whole story about the person

Head and neck
— scalp: bleeding, swelling, depressions
— eyes: vision, pupil size, redness, discharge
— ears: hearing, discharge (blood or clear fluid)
— nose: airway, bleeding, discharge
— mouth: bleeding, breath smell, teeth and gums, tongue, jaw
— throat: redness, ulceration, pus
— glands: neck, below jaw

Heart — pulse rate and regularity, blood pressure (judged by the force of the pulse and capillary filling; observe the speed at which the nail bed returns to a pink color after being blanched with pressure) — heart sounds (ear to chest) — peripheral circulation (warmth and color of the fingers and toes), ankle swelling

Chest — visible injury (bruising or fracture) — breathing movements and sounds (ear to the chest for air entry, wheeze and fluid crackling or bubbling)

Abdomen — quiet movement on breathing — scars from previous surgery, distension, swellings, genitals — tenderness, resistance to the examining hand, rigidity of muscle wall, masses or swellings, hernial openings

Pelvis and perineum — stability on pressing firmly on the hips — bruising between the legs, bleeding from the urethra

Muscles and joints — (for all limbs and joints) range of movement, pain, tenderness, swelling, deformity, power, tone, co-ordination, sensation, reflexes of all limbs and joints

Neurological — conscious level (Glasgow Coma Scale) and mental state, pupil size and reaction to light.

2 EQUIPMENT AND DRUGS

Before setting out on a journey to drive across the Sahara or sail the Pacific it would be wise to check the tool kit (and the machine) in order to make sure everything is present that might be needed to deal with a breakdown. For similar reasons the sections on Equipment and Drugs are included at the very start of this book so the reader may know what is available for dealing with the emergency at hand.

The first-aid kit (FA) contents will fit in a waterproof plastic box measuring 12x12x4cm (5x5x2"), the medical kit (Med), which is more comprehensive, in a box 24x16x6cm (9x6x3"). On an expedition much bulkier equipment and more drugs can be carried to base camp and the contents (Base) can be quite sophisticated, especially if a doctor is present.

Swiss Army Knife = SAK

Equipment

ITEM	F-A	MED	BASE
soap bar	*	*	
alcohol swabs		*	
Band-aids (assorted)	*	*	
Elastoplast strip 3"	*	*	
surgical adhesive tape 1"	*	*	
3"		*	
Steristrips	*	*	
moleskin	*	*	

ITEM	F-A	MED	BASE
bandage, elastic 3"	*	*	
knitted cotton 3"	*	*	
triangular		*	
safety pins	*	*	
gauze, sterile plain	*	*	
non-stick		*	
wound dressing #15		*	
paraffin tulle-graz		*	
Sofratulle	*	*	
gelatin foam		*	
scalpel blade #11	*	*	
#15		*	
forceps, thumb		*	
tweezers, eyebrow		*	
SAK	*		
scissors, dressing		*	
SAK	*		
forceps, locking (mosquito)		*	
syringes 3ml		*	
needles #25		*	
matches, waterproof	*	*	
luggage label	*	*	

ITEM	F-A	MED	BASE
wax pencil	*	*	
magnifying glass	*	*	
tongue depressor		*	
penlight	*		
thermometer, regular	*		
, low reading			*
flashlight			*
antiseptic concentrate			*
finger dressing, Tubegauz			*
head dressing, elastic net			*
paster of Paris/C-Cast			*
wire mesh splints			*
tincture of benzoin			*
needle driver			*
sutures 2/0 catgut			*
4/0 nylon			*
syringe 10ml			*
needles, hypodermic #20			*
surgical gloves			*
cervical collar			*
oral airway			*
nasopharyngeal airway			*

ITEM	F-A	MED	BASE
stethoscope			*
blood pressure cuff			*
ophthalmoscope			*
auroscope			*
Foley catheter			*
i/v drip set			*
i/v fluids			*
cricothyrotomy tube (sterile, wrapped)			*
dental forceps (upper)			*
(lower)			*
dental probe			*

Drugs

ITEM	STRENGTH	F-A	MED	BASE
D.1 ANALGESICS				
D.1.1 paracetamol	500mg tab		*	
D.1.2. naproxen	250mg tab		*	
D.1.3 codeine	15mg tab	*	*	
D.1.4. morphine	15mg tab		*	
	15mg/ml amp		*	
D.1.5. naloxone	0.2mcg/ml amp		*	

ITEM	STRENGTH	F-A	MED	BASE
D.2 ANTIBIOTICS				
D.2.1. cephalosporin	250mg tab		*	
	2g amp			*
D.2.2 co-trimaxazole	960mg tab		*	
D.2.3. metronidazole	250mg tab			*
D.3 ANTIHISTAMINES				
D.3.1. promethazine	25mg tab	*	*	
	25mg/ml amp			*
D.3.2 chlorpheniramine	4mg tab		*	
D.4 STEROIDS				
dexamethasone	0.5mg tab			
	20mg/ml amp			*
D.5 SEDATIVES				
D.5.1. lorazepam	1mg tab		*	
D.6 DIURETICS				
D.6.1. furosemide	40mg tab	*	*	
	10mg/ml amp			*
D.6.2. acetazolamide	250mg tab			*
D.7 CARDIO-VASCULAR DRUGS				
D.7.1 (= D.7.2) glyceryl trinitrate 0.5mg tab				*
D.7.2 adrenalin	1mg/ml inj			*

ITEM	STRENGTH	F-A	MED	BASE
D.8 RESPIRATORY DRUGS				
D.8.1. salbutamol	4mg tab		*	
D.8.1 salbutamol	puffer		*	
D.9 DIGESTIVE SYSTEM DRUGS				
D.9.1 aluminum hydroxide	500mg tab		*	
D.9.2 famotidine	40mg tab		*	
D.9.3. loperamide	2mg tab		*	
D.9.4 bisacodyl	50mg tab		*	
D.9.5 bismuth subgallate	200mg suppos			*
D.10 SKIN ANTISEPTICS				
D.10.1 povidone iodine	concentrate			*
D.11 SKIN APPLICATIONS				
D.11.1 betamethasone	0.1% oint			*
D.11.2 clotrimazole	1% cream			*
D.11.3 PABA sunscreen		*	*	
D.11.4 calamine				*
D.11.5 lip salve		*	*	
D.11.6 methyl salicylate	oint			*
D.12 EYES				
D.12.1 chloramphenicol	1% oint	*	*	
D.12.2 dexamethasone	0.1% oint		*	

ITEM	STRENGTH	F-A	MED	BASE
D.12.3 homatropine	2% drops		*	
D.12.4 local anasthetic	drops		*	
D.13 EARS				
D.13.1 chloramphenicol	1% oint		*	
D.14 NOSE				
D.14.1 phenylephrine	2.5% drops	*		
D.15 THROAT				
D.15.1 lozenges			*	
D.16 TEETH				
D.16.1 oil of cloves			*	
D.16.2 temporary filling			*	
D.17 LOCAL ANESTHETIC				
D.17.1 xylocaine 2%	20mg/ml vial		*	
D.18 ORAL REHYDRATION CONSTITUENTS				*

A mythology exists about the merits of particular drugs, encouraged by the habits of the prescriber and by advertising propaganda of drug manufacturers. Certain principles in recommending drugs are explained here; choice should be based on fact and good advice.

In the text drugs are given their scientific, generic names by which they are known world-wide. Prescribing the generic name is usually cheaper because drug companies load the cost of research and develoment onto their own brand names. It is also much safer because there can be no confusion over the name, which is the same in Tokyo or Timbuktu. When two drugs have similar action the cheaper is usually chosen; although cost is a factor in assembling a good medical kit it should not hamstring the choice if an expensive drug is markedly preferable. We are dealing in small quantities, and when they are needed only the best will do. If one drug has more than one action it is preferred. In order not to confuse a harrassed rescuer one well-tried drug, or possibly two, have been selected from each treatment category rather than offering many choices; many different antihistamines are available but promethazine and chlorpheniramine have stood the test of time. Medication once or twice daily is preferred because it is more likely to be remembered.

When recommending a drug or a piece of equipment I avoid repeatedly writing "if available". Included in my selection are such drugs and medical material as might reasonably be included in a wilderness medical kit, which should be comprehensive, compact and light. Most drugs are conveniently carried as pills or tablets rather than as liquids, which freeze, are bulky, and the bottles or ampules break easily. However, some drugs preferably are injected for speed of action, control, and to avoid vomiting; this book presumes that larger medical kits may include them, or that they may be found at base camp where they will necessarily require syringes and needles as well. The technique of intramuscular injection can be learned from any competent nurse and practiced on an orange, which has the form and consistence of skin. Intravenous injection requires more skill but millions of junkies have learned how.

Drugs are chosen to cover the widest spectrum of action, for example, the antibiotics cephalosporin and co-trimoxazole cover wide antimicrobial contingencies with few side-effects. If the person is sensitive to one, the other should be used. Sound hospital medicine is quite different to what can be practiced in the wilderness with a small medical kit and limited experience, and drugs may have to be chosen that would not be used in a more elaborate setting. Doses are given for an average-sized adult. Adjustments must be made for size and age. Children take roughly half the adult dose, infants a quarter. The possible side-effects of the drugs are spelled out. Pregnant women should beware of taking any drugs, unless well-advised.

Morphine and codeine are controlled drugs, that can only be prescribed by a registered physician under specific guidelines. When approached for small quantities of such drugs for their first-aid or medical kits, provided I know the person is competent to use the drugs safely, I prescribe a small amount (30 tablets maximum), writing the name of the person followed in red ink by "for expedition use only". The person is instructed that the name of the victim to whom the drugs are administered, the date, and the quantity must be written down each time and produced before any re-supplies will be prescribed. This seems a reasonable way to ensure that the law regarding controlled drugs is observed, although nothing specific is written in it concerning the dispensing of such drugs by non-medical people.

Each drug (D) is given a number; the first figure refers to the category, the second to its place within that group, for example (D.1.3) means the drug is in category 1, analgesics, and is number 3, codeine. When drugs are referred to in the text they are given this number and the rescuer must refer back to this chapter for details of action, dosage, and side-effects. When the choice is equal just the category number (D.1) is given. Thus this chapter deserves careful study before reading the rest of the text.

The specialized drugs mentioned in the Foreign Travel chapter are found only there and not in this general drugs section. When in the text is recommended a drug that does not appear in the medical kit it is enclosed thus [ergometrine]. Certain standard abbreviations are used throughout the book:

Rx:	drug treatment
s/e:	side-effects
i/m	intramuscular
i/v	intravenous
s/c	subcutaneous
s/l	sublingual
g	grams
mg	milligrams
mcg	micrograms
l	liters
ml	milliliters
tsp	teaspoon
tbsp	tablespoon

D.1   PAIN RELIEF — ANALGESICS
Pain is always unpleasant and often unnecessary because, with
adequate dosage of analgesics, most pain can be controlled. Pain
is very subjective and peoples' stoicism varies as does their
response to analgesics.

MILD ANALGESICS
Paracetamol will control most headache and mild muscular or
skeletal pain, and reduce fever; compared with aspirin, it causes
less irritation to the stomach, and possible bleeding, and fewer
sensitivity reactions. (Aspirin should be taken only in its enteric-
coated form that is released after passing through the stomach,
which is thus protected from its acid corrosion). Paracetamol has
little anti-inflammatory action.
   Naproxen one of many anti-inflammatory drugs, not related to
steroids, which are also analgesic; it may be taken in addition to
other stronger narcotic analgesics. Naproxen is useful for inflammatory conditions like arthritis, tendonitis, and bursitis.
   Compound analgesics containing aspirin or paracetamol mixed
with codeine or caffeine or both, have no advantages and are
expensive.

D.1.1 paracetamol
   Rx: 500mg-1g every 4 to 6 hours to maximum 4g daily
   s/e: rare hypersensitivity and skin rashes

D.1.2 naproxen
   Rx: 250-500mg twice daily
   s/e occasional stomach upset so take with food, and use
cautiously with sufferers of stomach ulcers, asthma, and aspirin
sensitivity; it may cause fluid retention at altitude

MODERATE ANALGESICS
Codeine serves several purposes; it relieves moderate pain, and can
be given together with paracetamol for increasing the analgesic effect of the latter. It suppresses cough, and reduces bowel motility
thus slowing diarrhea. It is the analgesic of choice in head injury
because pupil size and breathing are affected less than by morphine. Codeine is legally narcotic and potentially addictive, but
dependency is uncommon.

D.1.3 codeine phosphate

Rx: 10-60mg by mouth every 4 hours to a maximum 400mg daily

s/e: constipation, drowsiness, dizziness, alcohol enhancement

STRONG ANALGESICS

Morphine is a time-honored strong analgesic effective against severe pain; it causes euphoria. It is narcotic, causing sleepiness, and is also strongly addictive. It depresses breathing so should not be used when breathing is compromised, as in asthma and some chest injuries, and at high altitude. In head injury it depresses breathing and alters pupil size, which is an important diagnostic sign. A well-respected mountaineering and emergency physician says,

> " . . . all strong analgesics depress respiration; this effect is dose-related, as is the pain relief. Pain-killers don't "kill" pain. They need to be given until the conscious person says, with a big grin, "yes, it hurts like hell and I don't give a shit', not to a point of stupor."

Morphine constipates; it may cause nausea and vomiting, side-effects that can be lessened if it is combined with promethazine, which does not diminish the analgesic power and may even enhance it.

Morphine tablets [or the newer synthetic opioid buprenorphine] placed under the tongue, although bitter-tasting, are quickly and evenly absorbed; but swallowed morphine tablets are absorbed poorly from the stomach and the drug is broken down by the liver before it reaches its site of action in the brain. Hence the sublingual route is now preferred by many pain clinics, even though morphine has traditionally been given intravenously in small doses, repeated as often as needed. When given to a shocked person the injected drug can lie stagnant in the muscle because of poor circulation; when blood flow quickens, a slug of the drug is released suddenly and may depress breathing profoundly. Ideally the narcotic antagonist drug naloxone should be available in order to reverse respiratory depression.

Demerol is weaker than morphine and has no advantage so gets no space here.

D.1.4 morphine sulphate

Rx: 10-30mg maximum every 4 hours s/l, s/c, or i/m.

By i/v Rx 5mg every 5 minutes until pain is relieved and then repeated as frequently as needed to control pain.

s/e: respiratory depression, constipation, urinary retention, nausea, tolerance and dependance. Avoid in head injury, asthma, breathing difficulty, at high altitude, and with druggies.

D.1.5 naloxone, narcotic antagonist

Rx: 40-200 mcg i/v, and add 40 mcg every 2 minutes as needed to restore normal breathing; it can also be given i/m or s/c

s/e: nausea and vomiting

D.2 ANTIBIOTICS

Antibiotic drugs combat bacterial infections; virus illnesses are generally untreatable so antibiotics should be eschewed. Ideally bacteria should be grown in culture and their sensitivity ascertained before starting an appropriate antibiotic. However, in wilderness no such scientific accuracy is possible and a blunderbuss approach is in order, using an educated guess at which broad-spectrum antibiotic will be effective.

The only logical way to choose amongst the myriad antibiotics on the market is to take sound bacteriological advice and select two or three antibiotics in order to combat the widest range of organisms, with due consideration to cost and availability. Cephalosporins have superceded amoxycillin (a broad-spectrum penicillin which used to be the antibiotic of choice) because many organisms have become resistant to it. 5% of the population are penicillin-sensitive, but only 10% of penicillin-sensitive people are allergic to cephalosporin. 90% of Staphylococcus aureus, the universal organism of wound and soft tissue infections, and burns, all of which may be commonly encountered in wilderness, are resistant to amoxycillin whereas cephalospirin is effective against it. A new drug, ciprofloxacin, may soon become the blunderbuss antibiotic.

Cephalosporin is the name of a group of broad-spectrum antibiotics of which there are several to choose from, all with very similar actions, for example, cefaclor, cephalexin, cephradine. Hence the group name is offered rather than any single drug, for which advice can be taken from any doctor or pharmacist.

Cephalosporin is also very effective given i/v.

Cefalosporin is *bactericidal* and effective against group A streptococcus, Staphylococcus aureus, ampicillin-resistant Escherichia coli and Proteus mirabilis, Klebsiella pneumoniae, and Strep. pneumoniae — but ineffective against pseudomonas and Strep. fecalis.

Rx: against infections of skin and soft tissue, the middle ear, upper and lower respiratory tract (including streptococcal sore throat), and urinary tract.

Co-trimoxazole, a mixture of 5 parts sulphamethoxazole and 1 part trimethoprim, is the other antibiotic of choice for the breadth of its spectrum.

Co-trimoxazole is *bacteriostatic* and effective against Staph. aureus, H. influenzae, E. coli, klebsiella, enterobacter, Proteus mirabilis and vulgaris, Salmonella typhi and paratyphi, and shigella — but ineffective against Strep. fecalis and other streptococci.

Rx: against infections of burns, skin and soft tissue, bone and joints, the lower respiratory tract (bronchitis and pneumonia), and urinary tract; it is useful for bacterial diarrhea and in people who are allergic to penicillins and cephalosporins, though not if they are sulpha-sensitive. If a known doubly-sensitive person is on a trip tetracycline or erythromycin should be taken as a substitute.

Metronidazole (Flagyl) is active against anaerobic bacteria and protozoa, but has less antibacterial value than either cephalosporin or co-trimoxazole. It is well absorbed, giving high blood levels for a prolonged period. In the wilds far from help it would cope with persistent diarrhea of Entameba histolytica or Giardia lamblia, and with peritonitis following a ruptured appendix.

A full course of antibiotic usually lasts 5 to 7 days and should not be curtailed, but can be lengthened if the response is slow. Don't take alcohol with antibiotics. For convenience antibiotics are taken by mouth but in severe infections they are more effective i/v, though only sophisticated medical kits will carry them in this form.

D.2.1 cephalosporin

Rx: 250mg every 8 hours, doubled in severe infection

s/e: hypersensitivity and allergic symptoms of urticaria, rashes, nausea, vomiting, diarrhea, and in rare cases, anaphylaxis

D.2.2 co-trimoxazole
Rx: 1 double-strength (DS) tablet twice daily, doubled in severe infection

s/e: nausea, vomiting, rashes, and various blood disorders

D.2.3 metronidazole
Rx: 500mg every 8 hours

s/e: nausea, drowsiness, headache, rashes

D.3 ANTIHISTAMINES

Antihistamines dampen allergic reactions and ease hay fever, itching, skin rashes, vertigo and motion sickness; they are mildly hypnotic. They are used i/v in emergency treatment of severe allergic reactions but are of no value in asthma.

Promethazine is well-proven in alleviating nausea and vomiting; it can be given together with morphine, the analgesic effect of which is not diminished and may even be enhanced. It lasts up to 12 hours, and is quite sedating.

Chlorpheniramine is shorter-acting and less powerful, but is good for daytime use in treating allergies because it induces less drowsiness.

D.3.1 promethazine (Phenergan)
Rx: 25mg by mouth every 8 hours to maximum 150mg daily

s/e: drowsiness, headaches, urinary retention, dry mouth, blurred vision

D.3.2 chlorpheniramine
Rx: 4mg by mouth every 8 hours

s/e: less sedating than other antihistamines

D.4 STEROIDS

Dexamethasone (a powerful relative of prednisone) has widespread effects on the body and so should be used cautiously. It suppresses severe allergic reactions and may be effective in severe asthma, status asthmaticus, and acute hypersensitivity reactions like food and drug allergy and insect stings. In the wilds it could save the day for someone with an acute prolapsed disc or a severe gout attack, at least allowing them to walk to safety. It may reduce the brain swelling in cerebral edema of high altitude, and in trauma from head injury.

People taking steroids should wear a Medic-Alert bracelet or medallion and carry a card in their wallet with instructions on how to adjust their dose in case of emergency.

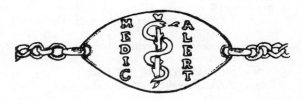

Medic-alert bracelet

D.4.1 dexamethasone (Decadron)

Rx: 4mg i/m or by mouth every 4 to 6 hours, or 10mg i/v, or i/m

Steroids are usually tailed off gradually, but can be stopped abruptly if the course has lasted less than 3 weeks.

s/e: steroids have many hazards, particularly in suppressing adrenal gland function and the normal inflammatory response; they should be taken under medical supervision.

D.5 SEDATIVES

Benzodiazepine drugs are useful hypnotics for insomnia or for long plane flights, and as sedatives in low doses for acutely anxious persons. When given i/v they may control epileptic seizures until the person can begin specific anti-epileptic medication. Benzodiazepines differ mainly in their length of action. Lorazepam is one of many available, being fairly quick of onset, short in action, and less cumulative than other benzodiazepines.

Promethazine (D.3.1) is a useful mild sedative.

D.5.1 lorazepam

Rx: 1 to 2mg at night, 0.5 to 1mg by day
s/e: drowsiness, dependency, habituation

D.6 DIURETICS

Diuretics promote urine flow and thus decrease edema by suppressing reabsorption of sodium by the kidney; coincidentally they lower blood pressure.

Furosemide is powerful and short-acting; only the smallest dose to get the required effect should be used, with caution. It treats edema of high altitude, of heart failure, pulmonary edema, and peripheral edema of the feet, ankles, and hands. Diuresis starts within 1 hour and is complete in 6 hours, so it is best taken in the morning because frequent peeing will disturb sleep. Used over a long time furosemide causes loss of potassium, which must be replaced as potassium tablets or by fruit juice.

Acetazolamide diminishes the incidence and effects of acute mountain sickness (AMS) and should be used at the first signs, but it is never a substitute for descent.

D.6.1 furosemide (Lasix)
Rx: 40 to 120mg daily by mouth, i/v not faster than 4mg/minute

s/e: potassium loss, dehydration, rashes, ringing in the ears

D.6.2 acetazolamide (Diamox)
Rx: 250mg 1 to 4 times daily

s/e: numbness and tingling of fingers, toes, face; dry mouth, makes beer taste foul

D.7 CARDIO-VASCULAR DRUGS
People with heart problems usually carry their own medications; the wilderness is no place to start cardiac drugs of unpredictable action and response.

Glyceryl trinitrate dilates blood vessels to the heart and relieves the chest pain of angina; it works within seconds and lasts less than an hour.

Adrenalin relieves acute asthma, severe allergic reactions and anaphylactic shock; it can be dangerous in older people because of causing heart irregularities.

Digoxin is risky to use and probably better left out of a medical kit.

D.7.1 glyceryl trinitrate
Rx: 0.5 to 1mg under the tongue and repeat in ½ hour if needed

s/e: throbbing headache, flushing, faintness

D.7.2 adrenalin
Rx: 0.5 to 1mg of 1:1000 solution by subcutaneous injection every 10 to 15 mins for 3 doses if needed
s/e: rapid, irregular pulse, anxiety, tremor, dry mouth, cold hands and feet.

D.8 RESPIRATORY DRUGS
Salbutamol is the safest bronchodilator drug and relaxes the tight wheezy breathing of asthma; it works rapidly when inhaled from an aerosol puffer but is more sustained and has more side-effects when taken by mouth. Beware of taking too much from the puffer because the drug is unevenly absorbed.

D.8.1 salbutamol (Ventolin)
Rx: 4mg by mouth every 6 to 8 hours; 2 puffs of aerosol every 6 to 8 hours; 0.25 to 0.5mg s/c or i/v in severe asthma
s/e: rapid pulse, headache, tremor

D.9 DIGESTIVE SYSTEM DRUGS
Antacids neutralize acid produced by the stomach and ease the discomfort of indigestion, gastritis, and the pain of peptic ulcer. They need to be taken frequently, after meals. Antacids bought in roll packets are convenient to carry in the pocket; tablets can be crushed to powder and made into a paste for quicker effect. Medication should go hand in hand with eliminating fatty or spiced foods, and avoiding nicotine, alcohol and coffee, all of which encourage gastric acid secretion.

D.9.1 aluminium hydroxide
Rx: 500mg tablets as needed
Acid-reducing drugs heal peptic ulcers; they block histamine receptors in the stomach, reduce gastric acid, and allow healing. They have no effect on bleeding ulcers.

D.9.2 famotidine
Rx: 40mg once daily at bedtime
s/e: diarrhea, skin rashes, dizziness

Gut-slowing drugs reduce motility and ease diarrhea. All narcotic drugs have this effect, often undesirable when used for pain relief.
Loperamide is poorly absorbed from the gut so remains longer where its action is needed; it can be used in parallel with codeine

(D.1.3), for greatest effect. Antibiotics may worsen diarrhea
because normal and necessary bowel organisms are killed as well
as harmful ones.

D.9.3 loperamide (Imodium)
Rx: 2mg every 8 hours
s/e: dry mouth, rashes

Laxatives of natural dietary roughage and fiber, like horses' bran
and whole wheat, along with fruit juice, especially of prune and
fig, may solve the problem more simply and safely than drugs.
  Motility-increasing drugs, if needed, act within 6 to 12 hours
and are fairly gentle purgatives which stimulate gut motility.

D.9.4 bisacodyl (Dulcolax)
Rx: 5 to 10mg by mouth after meals; by suppository 10mg
s/e: abdominal cramps, diarrhea

Piles and anal itching are helped by scrupulous toilet, washing
with soap and water after a bowel movement, avoiding constipation, and a bland astringent soothing cream. Sometimes hydrocor-
tisone (HC) and local anesthetic are incorporated into the
suppository.

D.9.5 bismuth subgallate (Anusol HC)
Rx: ointment or suppository twice daily

D.10 SKIN ANTISEPTICS
Antiseptic solutions cleanse and disinfect closed skin and open
wounds, but may cause sensitivity; they have no advantage over
washing with copious water and soap, hence are listed here only
for completeness. They are best carried as concentrate which can
be diluted with cooled boiled water.

D.10.1 povidone-iodine (Betadine)
Weakly antiseptic solutions can be made from crystals whose
bright color may contribute to their placebo effect; brilliant green,
gentian violet, potassium permanganate, methylene blue.

D.11 SKIN APPLICATIONS
Itching (pruritis) is often less bearable than pain and can drive a
person crazy; where possible treat the cause first. Topical antihistamines and local anesthetics are poorly effective and may

cause skin sensitization. Oral antihistamines are useful to subdue allergic skin rashes. Antibiotic creams are usually best avoided because most wounds and minor burns heal when left open to the air to dry; nothing supplants cleaning with soap and water. Systemic antibiotics are more effective than creams in many skin infections.

Steroid creams suppress skin inflammation, especially eczema, and relieve symptoms but do not cure the condition. Beware of rebound worsening on ceasing treatment. Side-effects may occur with long-continued use.

Clotrimazole is used against fungi, like monilia and tinea.

Sunscreens filter out the burning, erythema-producing parts of the ultra-violet spectrum.

D.11.1 betamethasone (Betnovate) 0.1% cream, a strong steroid
   Rx: apply thinly 2 to 3 times daily

D.11.2 clotrimazole (Canesten)
   Rx: apply 2 to 3 times daily, continuing for 1 to 2 weeks after the lesions have healed
   s/e: skin irritation and sensitivity

D.11.3 para-amino benzoic (PABA) esters
   Rx: apply 1 hour before exposure to sun and frequently thereafter

D.11.4 calamine ointment
   Rx: apply to itching skin

D.11.5 lip salve
   Rx: apply on under side of nose as well as lips

D.11.6 methyl salicylate muscle rub
   massage to produce soothing "deep heat"

D.12 EYES
Chloramphenicol is a broad spectrum antibiotic both for eye and ear, and ointment can be used in both.

Dexamethasone is a strong steroid for the treatment of iritis.

Homatropine, a mydriatic, dilates the pupil for about 24 hours and eases reflex iris spasm pain in corneal lesions.

Proparacaine local anesthetic acts within seconds and lasts a couple of hours; but it delays healing and should not be used over a long time.

D.12.1 chloramphenicol
  Rx: apply 1% ointment every 6 hours
D.12.2 dexamethasone
  Rx: apply 0.1% ointment every 6 hours
D.12.3 homatropine
  Rx: apply 2% drops twice daily
D.12.4 proparacaine (Ophthane)
  Rx: apply 1% drops as indicated

D.13 EARS
Chloramphenicol ointment put in the ear melts and flows through the canal as would drops; the same tube can be used for both ear and eye.
D.13.1 chloramphenicol
  Rx: apply 1% ointment every 6 hours

D.14 NOSE
Phenylephrine is a safe decongestant that takes effect within a minute and lasts 4 to 6 hours
D.14.1 phenylephrine 2.5% nose drops as needed

D.15. THROAT
At high altitude the cold dry atmosphere parches the throat so lozenges are needed in bulk.

D.16 TEETH
A lost filling could be a serious problem; insert oil of cloves into the cavity, then a temporary filling to stave off the pain.
D.16.1 oil of cloves
D.16.2 temporary filling

D.17 LOCAL ANESTHETICS
D.17.1 xylocaine 2% for injection

D.18 REHYDRATION SOLUTIONS
Fluid by mouth goes some way in helping redress upset body water balance resulting from shock, burns and dehydration (especially from diarrhea). Give sips of fluid enough to quench

thirst without causing vomiting.

The WHO formula is simple to make and contains most of the essential chemical components dissolved in 1 litre of boiled water:

glucose	20.0g =	1½ tsp honey, corn syrup
sodium chloride	3.5g =	½ tsp table salt
sodium bicarbonate	2.5g =	½ tsp baking soda
potassium chloride	1.5g =	¼ tsp or 2 cups of orange, apple, or other fruit juice.

Routes for giving medications

ORAL MEDICATIONS

Medicines can conveniently be taken by mouth in the form of tablets or capsules. Liquids, though better absorbed than pills, are not suitable for most wilderness medical kits because of weight, and the danger of breakage and freezing. Absorption from the stomach is uneven and takes a minimum of 2 hours, and an adequate therapeutic blood level may not be attained for 24 to 48 hours (especially in the case of antibiotics). Hence the onset of action is slow by mouth compared with the intravenous (fastest), subcutaneous (faster), or intramuscular (fast), routes. Oral medication is useless if the victim is unconscious, vomiting, or suffering from severe indigestion and nausea. However, in wilderness it is usually preferable to use pills. They are absorbed most quickly on an empty stomach, but sometimes because of acid constituents, must be taken with food. Some pills, for example morphine sulphate and glyceryl trinitrate, are absorbed well from the mucous membrane lining of the mouth, especially under the tongue, but the taste is bitter.

INJECTION TECHNIQUES

Before giving any injection read carefully, and ideally have a companion check, the label on the ampule or vial in order to make sure that the drug intended to be given is correct in name, strength, and dilution. Scrub hands thoroughly so all maneuvers will be as sterile as possible. If the drug is in an ampule, cover the neck with a piece of cloth or tissue, so any glass broken cannot accidentally cut your fingers. If the drug is in a rubber-capped vial, first clean the top with an alcohol swab. Assemble syringe and needle directly from their sterile packages taking care not to contaminate either. Draw a measured dose of fluid into the syringe; then hold it vertically, needle upwards, and expel any air bubbles. An orange has similar consistence to skin and can be used for practice in order to get the feel of thrusting a needle through skin, the thought of which imbues horror in many people.

Intramuscular injection (i/m); the sites of choice are:
— deltoid muscle over the upper outer arm a hands-breadth below the tip of the shoulder
— upper outer quarter of the buttock
— front of the thigh midway in a line between hip bone (iliac crest) and knee-cap.

Clean the skin with soap and water or an alcohol swab. Pinch the skin widely between thumb and fingers of one hand; holding the loaded syringe like a dart in the other hand, thrust it up to the hilt of the needle deep into muscle. Pull back on the plunger of the syringe to ensure the needle is not in a blood vessel; if blood returns into the barrel of the syringe withdraw the needle and start again. If clear, push steadily and slowly on the syringe plunger until the contents are completely evacuated. Withdraw the needle and clean the skin with the same swab, rubbing vigorously in order to spread the injected drug and to ease the discomfort of suddenly distending the tissues.

Subcutaneous injection (s/c): lax skin over muscle, such as the upper outer arm or abdomen, is suitable. Adrenalin is given s/c; morphine can be.
    Prepare as for i/m injection above. Pinch the skin only, and insert the needle at an angle until a "give" is felt as the point of the needle enters the fat layer just below skin but above muscle. Pull back on the plunger and inject slowly as above.

Intravenous injection (i/v); this route obtains the fastest action of the injected drug, and the technique can be learned with practice. But the effect of the drug is sudden and potent so the i/v route

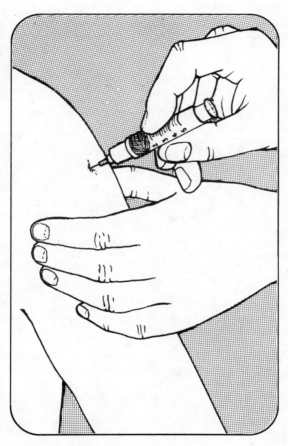

Intramuscular injection sites

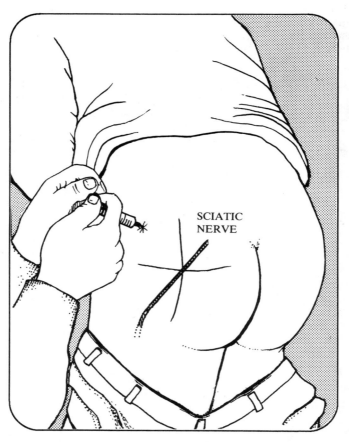

Intramuscular injection sites

should only be used by someone who fully understands the action and possible complications of the drug. The technique is summarized here in order to remind doctors who have spent time away from the sharp end of practice.

Obstruct the veins of the forearm and hand by tying some sort of tourniquet round the upper arm in order to make the veins stand out. This can be speeded by making the person clench and open a fist repeatedly, hang an arm over the side of the bed, immerse a hand in warm water or cover it with a hot, wet towel. Seek the largest vein on the back of the forearm for first choice, on the back of the hand next, in the crook of the elbow only if you can't find one elsewhere. Clean the skin with an alcohol swab where you intend to make the puncture. Stretch the skin over the vein tightly with one hand. Pierce the skin to the side of the engorged vein, angle the needle and advance it through the vein wall being careful not to pierce the opposite wall. Blood will return into the syringe if the needle is in place. Undo the tourniquet. Inject the required amount of drug slowly. Withdraw the needle, swab the site, and keep firm pressure for a minute. If the i/v site swells, the needle has probably punctured the vein and the drug has run into the tissues — it then has the effect of a s/c injection instead so leave it where it is.

3   AIRWAY BLOCK

Airway block occurs when the tongue falls back against the back of the throat (pharynx), or when saliva, blood, or vomit pool there; airway block can kill, so must be relieved immediately. However, any victim of severe trauma or heart attack who is not breathing is most likely dead, so only start resuscitation if there is some possibility of recovery and rescue.

Look, feel, listen

If breathing appears to have stopped bend over the person. Look for normal breathing with your eyes watching his chest and upper abdomen; feel for breath with your cheek against his mouth; listen with your ear against his nose. A partially blocked airway causes noisy breathing like someone snoring or croaking. The lips may be tinged blue (cyanosis) instead of their normal pink color, and froth may appear at the mouth. If breathing is obstructed chest movement is shallow and the spaces between the ribs are drawn inwards with each breath. Breathing sounds can be heard as well with your ear placed against his chest as by using a stethoscope.

> The structure and function of the tongue are crucial to understanding airway block. In quiet, normal breathing air passes through the nose; the mouth remains closed, almost completely filled by the tongue which lies well forwards against the teeth and hard palate. The tongue is fixed at its base to the lower jaw (mandible); when fully protruded only about one third of its total bulk is seen. The tongue normally stays forwards in the mouth, but while a person is lying face upwards asleep, or unconscious, the relaxed tongue falls back by gravity against the pharynx, partly shutting off the airway. As air slips past the tongue, it vibrates against the back of the throat sounding like snoring. The tongue of an unconscious person can form an almost air-tight block, like a cork, across the pharynx.
>
> An unconscious person may be able to vomit, but the laryngeal, cough, and swallowing reflexes that prevent food, water, blood, saliva and vomit from going down the wrong way, are suppressed. If inhaled, these substances irritate the lining membrane of the terminal sacs of the lung (alveoli) causing fluid secretions, which obstruct gas exchange between blood and air.

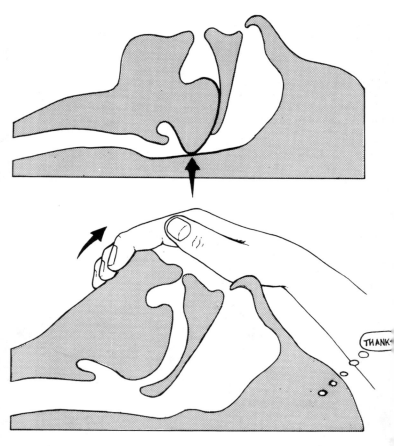

Airway and tongue anatomy

Inhaled air contains 20% oxygen which is carried by hemoglobin and gives saturated arterial blood its bright red color, making the lips pink. After combustion in the cells some of the oxygen is converted to carbon dioxide. Exhaled air contains only 16% oxygen, venous blood is unsaturated, and so the lips may be cyanosed and bluish.

After 4 minutes without oxygen the brain suffers irreparable damage. More brain cells die the longer oxygen is lacking, and they cannot regenerate as cells in some organs do. Although the victim may partly recover consciousness later, his brain will be permanently damaged.

Act: If breathing is obstructed unblock the airway with utmost speed. Turn the victim into the draining position, tilt the head, remove secretions, lift the jaw, insert a plastic airway, and fix the tongue. Hope he will not need an endotracheal tube, a cricothyrotomy or a tracheotomy — read on.

Draining position: Turn the victim on one side with his head lying lower than his body. Tilt the head slightly backwards (provided the neck is not injured) in order to straighten the neck and to avoid kinking the windpipe (trachea). Thus the tongue falls forward by gravity from the back of the pharynx so fluid can drain from the upper airway. This position has many names; coma, recovery, tonsil, but a single aim — drainage. If fluid has been inhaled through the vocal cords (larynx) into the lung, drainage has little effect and the victim may drown in his own juices.

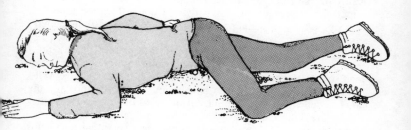

Draining position

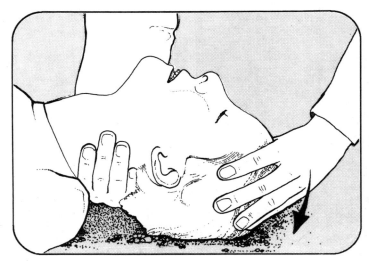

Head tilt

Head tilt: Tilting the head back slightly will straighten out the trachea, which may be kinked if the neck is flexed with the chin on the chest. One hand supports the neck, the other presses gently on the forehead. Even if the neck is injured it is more important to prevent the victim dying from suffocation than worrying about worsening a damaged neck, serious though that may be.

Finger sweep: Put a finger, wrapped in a piece of cloth, into his mouth and scoop out any obstructing solid matter such as vomited food, blood clot, or avalanche powder-snow. Don't remove well-fitting dentures. If the victim is conscious the teeth and jaws may be clenched tight; they should not be pried open because of the risk of breaking teeth. If conscious he can maintain his own airway anyway. The crossed-finger maneuver (see diagram) helps to hold the jaw open gently with a single hand, provided there is not much resistance.

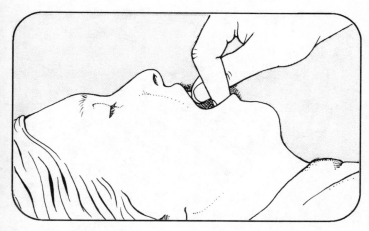

Crossed finger maneuver

Suck out: To remove fluid or secretions from the airway pass a flexible tube far back in the throat, suck on it and spit out the material. If secretions have pooled near the larynx this unpleasant task may be life-saving. Foot-operated suction pumps should be carried by rescue teams.

Jaw lift: Lift forwards the lower jaw, to which the tongue is fixed at its base, so the tongue moves with it and cannot fall back against the pharynx. It is easier to lift the jaw forward with the victim lying on his back, but the technique must also be learned in the draining position.

With three fingers of each hand widely spaced, grasp his jaw with the little finger curled behind the angle. Push it skywards rather than merely closing the upper and lower teeth together. This position is tiring but can be held for longer with the elbows resting on the ground. Holding the jaw with only one hand frees the other hand, but requires practice and some skill.

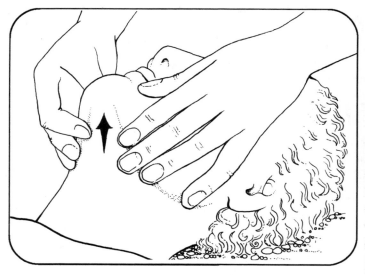

Jaw lift

Tongue fix: If the chin and tongue of an unconscious victim persistently fall back (for example, while being carried on a stretcher) and if you have no mechanical airway, thrust a safety-pin through the tip of the tongue, tie a piece of string to it, pull it firmly forwards and attach it to his belt; this apparently brutal action guarantees a clear airway. Should the victim regain consciousness the pin can be removed quickly leaving minimal damage.

Mechanical airways: Insert an airway if breathing remains obstructed notwithstanding all the above. A mechanical airway is not needed by a person who resists it, gags on it, or fights it, because the victim must be conscious enough to safeguard his own airway.

Oral airway: Carry a small, light, cheap plastic oral airway in a first-aid kit. The shaped end curves over the back of the tongue keeping open the space at the back of the pharynx. Open the

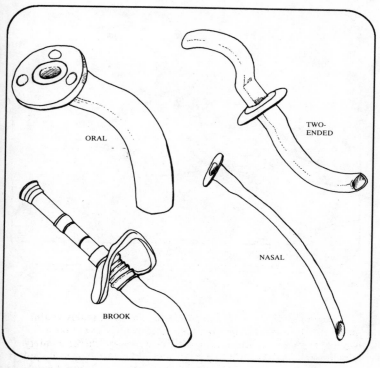

Mechanical airways

mouth wide, pull the tongue forwards, and insert the airway, moistened in order to slide more easily, with the curve pointing towards the roof of the mouth; then rotate it over the back of the tongue. The metal tooth guard prevents a half-conscious person biting it closed, and the flange stops it slipping down the throat.

2-ended oral airway: This makes mouth-to-mouth resuscitation less distasteful. An airway with a one-way valve and a cheek-guard is more efficient and can be attached to a self-inflating bag.

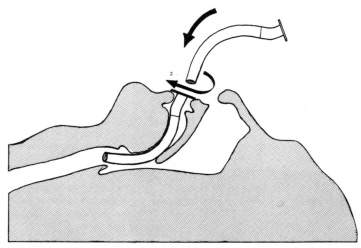

Inserting oral airway

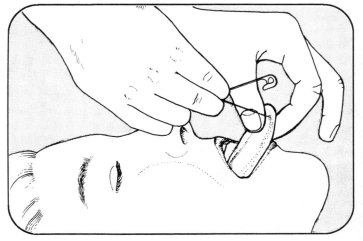

Tongue fix

NASO-PHARYNGEAL AIRWAY: Pass a well-greased tube about 15cm long through one nostril; gently and skillfully thread it backwards until the rubber flange lies against the nose (to prevent it being sucked down into the lung). Thus the end lies in the pharynx providing a clear airway past the tongue.

CRICOTHYROTOMY: A person about to die from unrelieved airway block can hereby be saved. Needless to say, such bold surgery requires courage, skill and good judgement. It is an acceptable procedure in dire emergencies in competent hands. Push a wide-bore #14 guage needle, or a knife blade, directly into the trachea through the cricothyroid membrane, which is easily found 1cm (½") below the prominence of the larynx (Adam's Apple) in the mid-line of the neck and above the cricoid cartilage. The thyroid gland and other vital neck structures are well lateral to the cricothyroid membrane, and the posterior ring of the cricoid cartilage should protect the esophagus behind. A hiss of air is released as the needle enters the trachea. A few puffs of air (or better, oxygen) may be enough to aerate the lungs and relax spasm of the vocal cords.

   A knife blade is inserted transversely through the skin over the cricothyroid membrane. The wound is spread with a knife handle or a dilator. A soft cuffed-tube inserted through the hole can be left in the trachea for 2 weeks or more. Pre-packed, sterile, diposable cricothyrotomy tubes can be bought commercially.

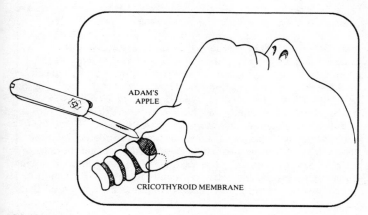

ADAM'S
APPLE

CRICOTHYROID MEMBRANE

Cricothyrotomy

ENDOTRACHEAL TUBE: The technique of passing an endotracheal tube
can be life-saving but should never be done by an untrained person.
Forcing a tube clumsily into the larynx causes spasm of the vocal cords,
which may only relax just before the victim is about to die. The skill of
endotracheal intubation once learned is never forgotten; rescue team
members should ask the anesthetist of the local hospital to teach them
how. Using a laryngoscope the tube is passed through the vocal cords
and lies in the trachea. It guarantees an open airway in all positions of
the head and neck during evacuation, and the modern, soft cuffed-tubes
can be left in place for 7-10 days before a formal tracheotomy need be
done. When the cuff surrounding the tube is inflated it seals off the
trachea and ensures nothing is inhaled into the lungs. It aerates the
lungs efficiently when attached to a self-inflating resuscitation bag,
preferably connected to a supply of oxygen.

   Tracheotomy is a surgical operation and should only be done in an
the operating room.

Absent breathing

RESCUE BREATHING
If the victim is unable to breathe despite an open airway, blow
oxygen into the lungs urgently — but only if there is a reasonable
chance of recovery and rescue. If he does not start breathing on
his own after half an hour the rescuer should stop resuscitation
(unless expert help is expected imminently) because his efforts are
fruitless and will be exhausting, imperiling his own retreat.

Mouth-to-mouth: The rescuer's own nasty expired breath,
although not as good as pure air, still contains 16% oxygen,
enough to change the victim's color from blue to pink. Turned on
his back is an easier position to do mouth-to-mouth than lying on
one side. Tilt the head. Wipe away debris and secretions in his
mouth. Place your mouth over his mouth and exhale fully into his
mouth while pinching his nose to stop air escaping. Watch his
chest, which will rise if the lungs are being adequately inflated;
about ¼ to ½ litre of air should be shifted with each breath.
Then remove your mouth; the elasticity of his own lungs will expel
the air. One breath every 4 to 6 seconds is ample. If his mouth is
injured breathe into his nose instead, holding his lips closed the
while.

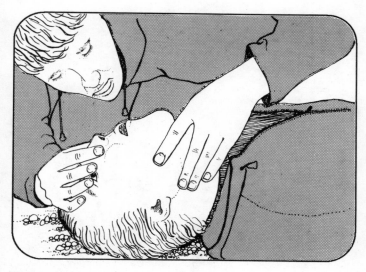

Mouth-to-mouth

SELF-EXPANDING HAND-INFLATED BELLOWS: Air is sucked through a valve at one end and expelled at the other. Inflation is easier work than mouth-to-mouth breathing and can be continued for longer. The bellows can either be attached to a face mask over the nose and mouth, or be connected to a mechanical airway.

Choking

The victim of choking from airway block caused by a foreign body grasps his throat, goes blue in the face and cannot speak.

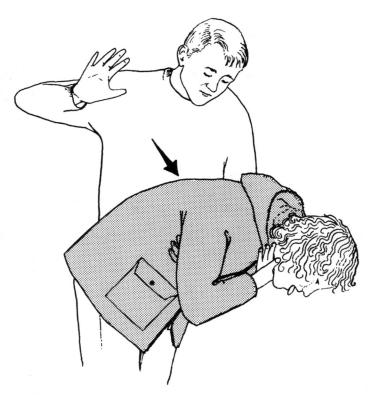

Back blows

Act: *Strike 4 sharp blows* rapidly with the heel of the hand in between his shoulder blades while supporting his breastbone (sternum) with your other hand. Open his mouth with one hand. Grasp his jaw and pull it forward. Sweep the index finger of your other hand as far back in the throat as possible and hook out any foreign material.

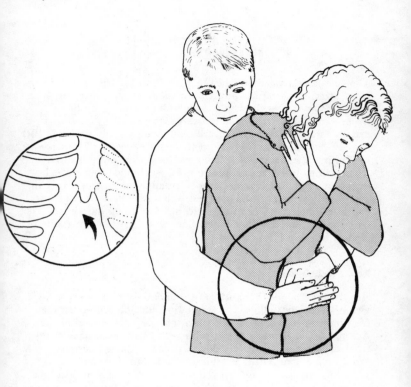

Heimlich Maneuver

Abdominal (or chest) thrusts (Heimlich maneuver) stand behind the victim, wrap your arms around him and grasp with one hand the closed fist of your other hand placed over the upper abdomen or lower chest. Give 4 thrusts strong enough to force air out of the lungs and to dislodge the obstruction, but not so violent as to rupture an internal organ.

4 HEART STOP (Cardiac Arrest)

The commonest cause of heart stop, even in the wilderness, is heart attack (myocardial infarction); the heart can also stop after severe trauma, near-drowning, a lightning strike or deep hypothermia. In a remote area heart stop caused by trauma is usually fatal. A summary of cardio-pulmonary resuscitation (CPR) is given here because it is one of the skills expected of all first-aiders, but the chance of it being successful in wild places far from help is nearly zero. Even in a fully equipped and staffed emergency room the success rate is usually reckoned at less than 5%. For this reason I am tempted to banish this section to the end of the book and print it small, but fear of an outcry from enthusiastic "hands-on" rescuers has persuaded me reluctantly to leave it in place.

Look, feel, listen

Absent pulse or heart sounds: Feel the carotid pulse in the victim's neck by sliding your finger tips into the groove between his windpipe (trachea) and the neck muscles at the level of the Adam's Apple (larynx). Listen with your ear pressed against the front of his chest to the left side of the breastbone (sternum); the heart sounds like a distant "lub-dup, lub-dup, lub-dup".

Feeling the radial pulse at the wrist is notoriously misleading; the rescuer's cold fingers searching for it under tight anorak cuffs may get the false impression that the heart has stopped. Alternatively feel in the groin for the femoral pulse, found halfway between the pubic bone and the wing of the pelvis (iliac crest).

Unconsciousness: The victim looks deathly pale and does not respond to command or pain. His pupils slowly dilate and do not constrict to the stimulus of light.

Absent breathing: Place your ear near his mouth. Listen and feel for movement of air.

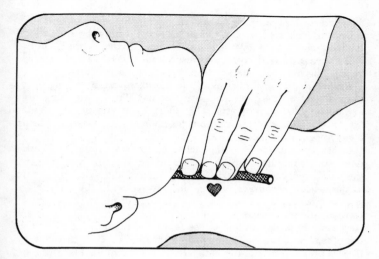

Carotid-artery Pulse

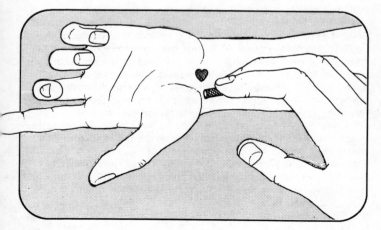

Radial-artery Pulse

Act: Irreversible brain damage occurs after the heart and breathing have stopped for 4 minutes so CPR must be started immediately to have any chance of success. If the victim is cold and appears dead always try to resuscitate and re-warm him because he may be suffering from hypothermia instead.

Rescue Breathing: Start mouth-to-mouth rescue breathing immediately with 4 quick, full breaths, not allowing the lungs to deflate fully between breaths. One sharp blow with the clenched fist on the middle of the sternum may sometimes restart the heart; if not, begin chest compression without ado.

Chest compression: Lay the victim horizontal, or slightly head down (but never head up) on a hard, flat surface in order to get the best gravity feed for blood to the brain. Later raise his feet on a rucksack to encourage venous blood to return to the central circulation. Kneel beside him, feel the edge of his rib cage, and run your fingers upwards until they meet the notch where ribs and sternum join in the middle of the lower chest. Place the heel of the other hand two finger-breadths above the notch with your fingers pointing across the long axis of the sternum. Place your free hand on top of the hand on the sternum so the fingers of both hands are parallel; fingers can be extended or interlocked but they should not rest on the chest.

Lock your elbows straight with shoulders positioned over your hands. Press down on the heels of your hands vertically, smoothly, and with sufficient force to depress the sternum 4 to 5cm in order to squeeze the heart enough to pump blood to the brain. Some ribs may fracture but this is not serious and can be dealt with later. Release the pressure completely after each compression in order to allow the heart to refill, but do not lose contact with the sternum. Compress the chest regularly and evenly.

Single rescuer: 15 to 2 sequence. Compress the chest 15 times, faster than once a second. Then give 2 quick, full rescue breaths lasting 4-5 seconds without allowing him time to exhale fully between breaths. Feel the cartoid pulse occasionally to check that heart compression is being effective and to see if the heart has restarted on its own.

2 rescuers: 5 to 1 sequence. Compress the chest once every second while an assistant does rescue breathing, giving a swift breath at

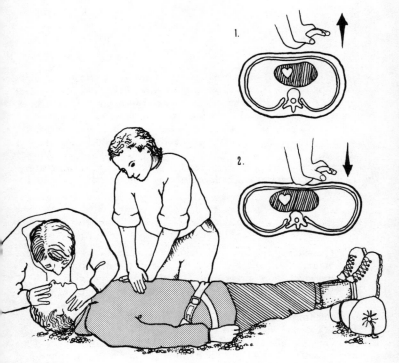

Chest compression

the up-stroke of every 5th compression without interrupting
compressions. Team-work and good timing are essential and need
practice.

Once started continue CPR until spontaneous heartbeat and
breathing have returned. The victim becomes warmer; blue lips,
pale skin and mucous membranes change to pink; and large
dilated pupils return to normal. Continue to watch him closely
because he may relapse. CPR is very hard work and ½ hour is
about the longest most people can manage on their own. If the
heart has not restarted within this time it probably never will.

5   HEAD INJURY

Generally speaking, bad head injuries tend to get worse and die, not-so-bad head injuries tend to get better. Less than 1% of head injuries need surgery; those that do, need it at once. Do not be tempted to interfere and risk worsening things. A Swiss Army knife or the pick of an ice-axe wielded in the field by a surgeon could be life-saving; in unskilled hands they would be lethal weapons.

Prevent the victim dying of, or being harmed by, other causes, the most important of which are airway block, neck injury, and bleeding.

Airway block

Snoring, rattling breathing is a sign of a blocked airway, not of head injury. Turn the victim on his side in the draining position with the head slightly downhill. Don't leave him lying on his back for fear of worsening a neck injury, because his tongue will sink backwards by gravity, block the airway and kill him. Also vomit or blood from an associated face or nose injury may trickle down the back of the throat and be inhaled. Hold the jaw forward and insert an oral airway. If the victim is deeply unconscious, or if his face is badly smashed, simply holding the jaw will probably not keep the airway open.

> Insert a naso-pharyngeal tube which has the advantage of by-passing an injured mouth. This difficult procedure can be done without direct vision. If the mouth is unharmed pass an endotracheal tube using a laryngoscope. If neither method is possible a cricothyrotomy may be necessary to prevent suffocation.

Neck injury

A victim of a head injury may also have injured his neck. Examine him carefully, avoid unnecessary movement, put on a cervical collar, and strap him to an improvised spinal board.

Bleeding

The scalp and face bleed profusely and alarmingly but such bleeding is a poor indication of the gravity of the head injury.

SCALP: Wash and clean with plenty of water and, if necessary, cut away some hair in order to get a better view and gain access to the scalp. Press firmly over the wound with a dressing pad — any cotton material placed on top of a sterile gauze square usually suffices to stop bleeding. Do not remove the first blood-soaked dressing because fresh clot will be disturbed, just add more dressings on top as needed. Usually scalp wounds heal well without suturing. For an open skull wound, or a suspected depressed fracture, make a dough-nut dressing, or a ring pad that presses around the wound edge on undamaged skull while leaving the center without pressure.

TEMPORAL ARTERY LACERATION: A minor cut over the temple area can sever the temporal artery which runs close under the skin over the skull, felt 2cm above and in front of the pinna of the ear. Sometimes the cut end spurts and can be seized with forceps and tied; otherwise pressure will have to suffice.

FACE: Wounds heal well but they demand accurate apposition of the edges in order to get the best scar, so use Steristrips or Butterflies to hold the edges together. A plastic surgeon can tidy up the scar later.

When the face is badly smashed with lacerations around the mouth, a fractured jaw and dislodged teeth, the airway is threatened and must be safe-guarded with an artificial airway, or best, with an endotracheal tube.

The victim of head injury may be conscious, in which case he can answer questions that will help make a diagnosis, or unconscious, when he will need to be cared for completely.

The unconscious person

After dealing with the life-threatening conditions above, attend to the following:

Restless behaviour: may result from brain disturbance, pain, or a full bladder; the victim may need restraining.

Pain: Rx: codeine (D.1.3). Do not use morphine, which depresses breathing, alters consciousness, and constricts the pupils thereby disguising a vital observation.

Bladder: a bursting bladder causes an unconscious person to thrash about in bed. Encourage him to pee by stroking the inside of the thighs accompanied by the sound of water flowing from one cup to another.

If this fails do a suprapubic stab with a wide-bore needle. When the bladder is full repeated stabs are safer and less likely to result in infection than attempting to catheterize in unclean conditions.

Feeding: an unconscious person will be unable to feed himself and, if neglected over several days, may become starved and dehydrated.

Pass a naso-gastric tube with a funnel attached by which he can be fed directly into the stomach. Plain water is better than nothing. Desist if there is any suspicion of basal skull fracture because the tube may penetrate through the fracture into the brain.

Eyes: lubricate with any eye ointment to prevent the cornea developing ulcers from drying by exposure to the air.

Skin: turn him every 2 hours to prevent bedsores, that readily become infected causing blood poisoning (septicemia) — a common cause of death in head injuries. Scrupulous attention to bowels and to hygiene of the perineum will prevent soiling by feces, which causes the skin to become raw and liable to pressure sores.

MECHANISM OF HEAD INJURY

Brain is composed of semi-solid nerve tissue suspended in cerebro-spinal fluid (CSF), which cushions movement of the brain within the skull — a rigid, protective box. CSF circulates between a layer of tissue (arachnoid), covering the brain, and another lying against the skull (dura). Blood vessels in the space between brain and arachnoid, and between skull and dura, are liable to be torn in a severe head injury. Spilled blood has no means of escape and gathers in spaces between the covering layers causing pressure to rise inside the skull.

Primary brain injury, caused at the moment of impact by displacement, distortion, and stretching of brain within the skull dictates the final outcome of the head injury.

Skull fracture, may be linear, comminuted into small fragments, depressed below the surrounding skull or through the base of the skull. A fracture may be closed or open (compound) and is superimposed on the primary brain injury. When open the brain communicates with the outside either directly, or via the nose or ears, where CSF leakage can be seen as drops of clear fluid. If infection enters the consequences may be lethal; a sulpha antibiotic is preferred because it crosses the blood-brain barrier; otherwise Rx co-trimoxazole (D.2.2).

TYPES OF BRAIN DAMAGE

Concussion: A trivial blow on the head causes the brain to swirl round, nerve pathways are deranged, and the victim falls unconscious briefly. After resting he may recover quickly and completely. Someone "knocked-out" may be unconscious from a few seconds up to several minutes. The speed at which he regains normal consciousness is a good indicator of the severity of the injury and of the final outcome. He may forget the impact itself but will probably remember events up to the accident. Then follows a measurable period of forgetfulness (post-traumatic amnesia) which is important because an injured person may feel fine and set off alone, without recollection of the accident or of his whereabouts. He may lose his way, or worse, relapse and collapse owing to pressure from slow, hidden bleeding gathering within the skull. Anyone who has lost consciousness from a head injury, for however short a time, should not be allowed to go unattended, even if he considers his injury trivial.

Contusion, laceration, and local damage: With more severe trauma specific areas of the brain may be bruised or mangled. The brain has well-defined areas that control limb movement, speech and sensation. The right half of the brain controls the left side of the body and vice-versa. Local damage can cause irritation of the brain with fits of twitching of the opposite limbs; these may spread into general grand mal epileptic seizures during which the victim may die from airway block. Occasionally the limbs are paralysed on the opposite side of the body. Recovery is slow.

Clot compression: Concussion may follow a trifling knock on the head or severe intracranial bleeding. The victim improves and appears quite normal a short while later (lucid interval) and he may even continue the expedition. Continued bleeding (extradural hemorrhage) or swelling of the brain itself causes pressure to rise within the rigid skull with subsequent compression of the brain. He complains of headache; then he relapses, becomes more drowsy and slips into coma. The victim will die unless the blood under pressure is released quickly by a surgeon drilling a trephine hole in the skull. Brain damage from compression is permanent because cells of the outer layer of the brain cortex die, unlike cells in other parts of the body which can regenerate.

Rx: dexamethasone (D.4.1) may reduce the pressure somewhat. Surgery is the best treatment so rescuers must evacuate the victim fast.

Severe, diffuse injury: The climber is deeply unconscious from the time of injury and unable to keep an open airway. He may be lax or stiff. Unless prevented he may roll about in a purposeless manner and fall again. If the airway is protected he may recover slowly over several months.

Observe & record

After taking immediate steps to prevent the victim of head injury dying, the biggest contribution to the final outcome will be accurate hourly recording of changing trends in his level of consciousness and of clinical progress. Your notes may help the surgeon, who will see him for the first time some hours later, to decide whether to operate immediately in order to relieve pressure from bleeding within the skull (cerebral compression). If observations are not written down during the tumult of the rescue, they won't be remembered accurately enough afterwards to be of value.

ASK: In addition to the usual history ask these specific questions from the victim if conscious, or if not, from a witness:

— Details of the accident: exact time, length of fall, falling objects, roped or helmeted?
— Unconscious? if so, for how long?
— Convulsions?
— Alteration in victim's behavior or level of consciousness?
— Hypothermia at the site of the accident?

Look, feel, listen

Unconsciousness may be the result of convulsions, before or after the injury, caused by illness unrelated to the head injury. Look for a Medic-Alert bracelet or neck-chain medallion which may tell of known illnesses (epilepsy, diabetes) and current medication.

The Head: Remove any hat or helmet in order to inspect the whole head. Slip a hand under the neck to see if blood has pooled there. Wash wounds with soap and water and remove blood clot and hair in order to display the depths of the wound. Look for a fracture. Never probe a wound and risk introducing infection, or even penetrating the brain through an open skull fracture. A large, boggy swelling under the scalp, or the absence of an open wound suggest blood collecting at the site of a skull fracture. Pieces of foreign material must be removed before dressing the wound.

Clear fluid oozing or dripping from the nose (rhinorrhea) or ears (otorrhea) suggests leakage of cerebro-spinal fluid from a fracture of the base of the skull. Bleeding from the nose or ears, when not caused by obvious external injury, may also come from inside the skull. Both are signs of grave injury and need urgent surgical attention.

Rx: antibiotics (D.2) in maximum doses.

Conscious level: The Glasgow Coma Scale is used internationally to estimate the conscious level and replaces vague, confusing terms of yore like "stupor" and "black-out". Noting the scale over several hours will show if the conscious level is becoming lighter and approaching normal, or is deepening because of increasing pressure on the brain from within the skull owing to bleeding or swelling.

THE GLASGOW COMA SCALE

Eye opening (E)	
spontaneous	4
to command	3
to pain	2
nil	1
Best Motor response (M)	
obeys command	6
localizes pain	5
withdraws from pain	4
abnormal flexion (to pain)	3
extensor response (to pain)	2
nil	1
Best Verbal response (V)	
oriented & converses	5
disoriented & converses	4
inappropriate words	3
incomprehensible	2
nil	1

Levels of response (E + M + V)
  total 8 to 7 = will probably survive
  total 6   = doubtful outcome
  total 5 to 4 = will almost certainly die
  total 3   = nearly dead

Eyes: The pupil of an unconscious person, whose brain is being compressed by an enlarging pool of blood, dilates on the side of the clot and tells the surgeon on which side to drill a trephine hole. The pupil fails to respond by constricting to light because the occulomotor nerve, which controls pupil size, becomes stretched and eventually paralysed. If the pressure is not relieved the opposite pupil becomes paralysed and fails to constrict to light. Two fixed dilated pupils indicate the victim is almost surely dead. If one pupil is bigger than the other in an awake, alert

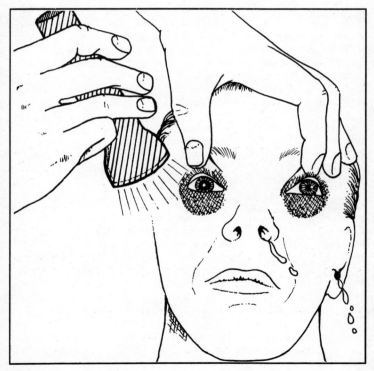

Head injury

person it may be because the light is coming more strongly from one side, the pupil may have been like that since birth, or as the result of a blow on the eye (traumatic mydriasis).

If the victim blinks when a hand is waved close in front of his eye — a visual threat — the visual pathways to the brain are intact. A wisp of cotton wool touching the cornea should elicit a reflex blink.

OPHTHALMOSCOPE EXAMINATION Papilledema occurs in advanced cranial pressure. Retinal hemorrhages suggest the presence of blood in the sub-arachnoid space owing to sudden increase in intra-cranial pressure from the primary brain injury.

Pulse, breathing, & temperature: Raised pressure inside the skull causes the pulse to slow and blood pressure to rise — as opposed to shock in which the pulse quickens and blood pressure falls. Breathing becomes irregular and periodic (Cheyne-Stokes). The temperature of the victim of a severe head injury may soar to 41°C (106° F), or more because of a disturbed heat-regulating center. Cool him vigorously with cold water, ice or snow.

Sensation & Power: Loss of feeling to light touch with a pin, or numbness and tingling, may indicate damage to the peripheral nerves, spine, or brain. Progressive one-sided weakness suggests localized brain damage. The limbs may become partially or completely paralysed.

Consider other causes of coma in an unconscious person who tells no story, nor shows any sign of, head injury. Look for a Medic-Alert bracelet or medallion. But remember that the victim may also have struck his head while falling unconscious for other reasons.

6   SPINAL INJURY

All head injury victims with altered consciousness, as well as those people complaining of neck pain after injury, should be treated as having a fracture and/or dislocation of the spine until proved otherwise — 15% will have such injuries. Care of the airway is paramount so, it is in order to gently move the neck by head tilting and jaw lifting. First-aiders are often brain-washed against moving under any circumstance the victim with a neck injury, resulting in inadequate treatment of life-threatening injuries. Airway block kills far more often than neck injury itself.

Neck fracture and/or dislocation

Suspect a fracture and/or dislocation if the victim has been, or still is, unconscious; fell from a height and injured his head or face (20% have associated spinal injury); suffers neck pain and tenderness, or holds his neck in an abnormal position; complains of loss of feeling, or tingling and numbness, in the hands or arms; or is unco-operative and mentally changed as a result of head injury, shock or even alcohol.

Act: take the victim with all speed but without further damage to a hospital where he can be X-rayed, accurately diagnosed and given expert treatment. In the meantime do the best you can and make sure he does not die from causes other than the neck injury. If the spine is fractured and/or dislocated the injury will probably be so severe you are unlikely to worsen the damage; the paraspinal muscles go into rigid spasm splinting the neck so any subsequent displacement will be minimal compared to the initial force that caused the injury. However, bruising and swelling may spread upwards in the spinal cord affecting progressively higher levels.

If the victim is awake and alert and wants to move his neck let him do so; the main reason for splinting the neck is so the rescuers cannot unwittingly shift an unstable fracture and/or dislocation making it worse. Similarly, if he wants to and can walk,

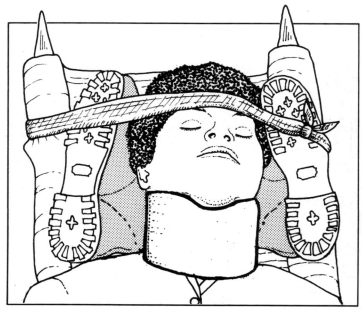

Neck injury—collar and head strap

let him do so. If he cannot move himself he may have to be moved to a safer place to be resuscitated or splinted to a spinal board.

Splinting: Make a collar of tightly-rolled clothing or newspaper, aluminum foil, or a well-padded wire splint about 10cm wide, and secure it around his neck with tape so it fits snugly under his chin. Do not try to correct any deformity of his neck. Splint it with 2 rolls of clothing on either side of the head, or with a pair of boots soles outwards uppers under the neck. Strap or tape round the forehead so the head is splinted to the board.

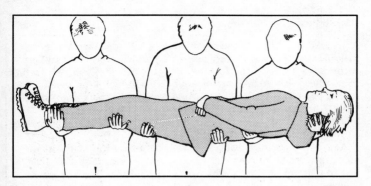

One piece move

Moving: Before moving the victim give a strong pain-killer.
Move him in one piece to avoid increasing the displacement of any
dislocated vertebrae. One rescuer holds the head, one the legs,
and another the body; all move together on command so the
victim's head does not twist on his shoulders, nor his body on his
pelvis. A collar alone will not entirely stabilize the neck, but a
spinal board will do so.

Spinal board: Lay the victim flat on a spinal board which can
be improvised from two pack-frames lashed together, or on a
stretcher. Tie him so firmly to the board that he cannot move and
yet the board can be tipped over in case of vomiting.

AIRWAY
Naso-tracheal intubation is preferable if the victim is breathing; if not
do a cricothyrotomy. A naso-gastric tube reduces the chance of vomiting
and aspiration, and prevents distension of the stomach from gastro-
intestinal ileus which often accompanies spinal injury.

Rx: codeine (D.1.3). Avoid narcotic drugs like morphine which
depress breathing and could kill someone whose chest muscles are
paralysed.

dexamethasone (D.4.1) may decrease spinal cord swelling.

Back injury

A severe back injury, though unlikely to kill someone outright, may paralyse from the waist down. A paralysed person may be surprisingly tranquil; he feels as though cut in half with no feeling below the waist. At the site of injury he will feel pain, which radiates round his middle from that level and shoots down his legs. If he can move fingers and toes, and if he can feel light touch, no nerves are damaged. But do not move the limbs actively or you may cause further injury.

Act: if the victim is conscious and in full control of his airway, and can walk by himself, let him do so. If he cannot walk he will probably be most comfortable lying on his back on a stretcher.

If he is unconscious tie him firmly to a spinal board or stretcher which can be tipped on its side should he vomit. Loosen tight clothing. Pad bony prominences between the knees and ankles, and body hollows especially behind the neck. Bandage his legs together so he may be more easily moved in one piece.

If he is *paralysed*, turn him every hour. A paralysed person cannot feel pain or the normal sensations of touch, pressure and temperature. He will lie quite still. Pressure on the skin, normally relieved by shifting body position will hamper blood flow locally causing painless sores which can develop in less than an hour and take weeks to heal, especially if infected. Make sure he is not lying on crumpled bedding and clothing. Remove from his pockets hard objects, which cause uneven pressure. If incontinent of bladder or bowels keep him clean and dry with regular hygiene and, if possible, an indwelling catheter.

MECHANISM OF SPINAL INJURY
The spine's 24 vertebrae form a column between skull and pelvis. Forces are transmitted through bony vertebral bodies behind which lie vertebral arches that form a protective tunnel for the spinal cord. Nerves to the arms leave the spinal cord highest, then those for the trunk, and finally those for the legs. The spine can bend and twist by way of many vertebral joints. Semi-solid discs between the vertebrae act as washers to cushion stress forces. Ligaments and powerful muscles stabilize the entire length of column.

A fractured or dislocated vertebra may damage nerves by pressure and sheering. The higher the spinal cord injury the more extensive will be the damage to nerve pathways below that level. If the cord is cut across in the neck all four limbs, chest and abdomen will be paralysed

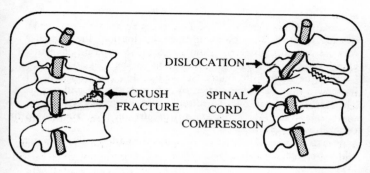

Vertebral fracture

(quadriplegia); if the injury is in the middle of the back only the legs and bladder will be affected (paraplegia). Damage to the brain paralyses the opposite side of the body because nerve pathways cross in the brain stem (hemiplegia).

Other spinal problems

WRY NECK (acute torticollis)
The neck and head are pulled towards one shoulder because neck muscles go into tight spasm, usually on waking after sleeping in an awkward position.

Act: apply ice packs alternating with heat and gentle massage.

NECK SPRAIN (whiplash)
Whiplash can occur after a fall without visible damage to either head or neck. Severe neck pain may last several months.

Rx: analgesics (D.1), cervical collar.

BACKSTRAIN (lumbago)
The paraspinal muscles go into painful spasm in order to splint the vertebral joints.

Rx: analgesics (D.1), rest, local heat, avoid heavy lifting or bending.

SLIPPED DISC (sciatica)
A prolapsed intervertebral disc may press on spinal nerve roots causing pain and tingling along their distribution: the arms if a cervical vertebra, the legs if lumbar. Sciatica is pain felt in the leg along the course of the sciatic nerve; in the buttock, down the back of the thigh, into the calf and possibly as far as the heel or foot. Pain may be accompanied by loss of sensation and weakness. The straight leg can only be raised 30° to 40° from the horizontal.

Rx: analgesics (D.1), rest on a firm surface, evacuate if signs of nerve pressure are present.

dexamethasone (D.4.1) in a desperate situation only, it might allow a person to walk out to safety.

PERIPHERAL NERVE INJURIES
Most will return to normal once the offending stimulus is removed.

Lateral femoral cutaneous nerve: a tight waist belt may cause loss of feeling in the upper outer thigh.

Brachial plexus palsy: tight pack-sack shoulder straps cause pressure on the brachial plexus. The whole arm may go numb and feel weak. If the upper spinal cord only is affected sensation is lost over the tip of the shoulder, the upper outer arm and the forearm. The elbow cannot be moved outwards nor can the hand rotate.

Anterior tibial compartment "shin splints": over-use causes pain in the muscle lateral to the ridge on the shin bone (tibia). The foot cannot be flexed upwards so on walking the foot drops and drags, which can be permanent. Sensation is diminished in a small area on adjacent sides of the big toe and the second toe. This is surgical emergency.

7   CHEST INJURY

In a serious accident both head and chest may be injured, but the chest injury may pass unnoticed because of the more obvious head injury. However both head and chest must be examined because injuries to either may be fatal — the chest often more rapidly so than the head.

The chest may be crushed (closed injury) by a tumble onto rock or a tree, a falling stone, or by sudden tightening of a rope. It may be punctured (open injury) by a spike of rock or the pick of an ice-axe.

Act: before attempting a diagnosis, keep open the airway; seal the open wound with a thick, impermeable dressing like paraffin gauze, plastic kitchen wrap or plastic bag taped to the skin all

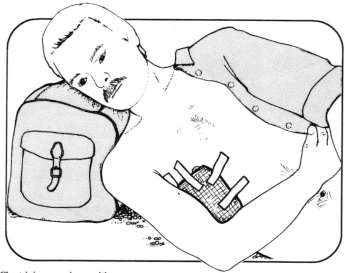

Chest injury nursing position

round in order to prevent escape or entry of air; splint the chest
by binding the victim's arms, bent at the elbow, across his chest.
Turn him to lie on the injured side with the weight of his own
body splinting the chest wall which may be unstable. Use clothes
as extra padding and to add pressure.

> If the airway remains blocked and if cyanosis persists despite the above,
> consider endotracheal intubation or cricothyrotomy and artificial
> ventilation.

Rx: morphine (D.1.4) may be needed to control pain and allow
deep breathing. By tradition narcotics are not used in chest injury
because they depress respiration; but by relieving pain most people
with chest injury breathe better, so be judiciously bold. Morphine
can always be reversed with naloxone (D.1.5).

antibiotic (D.2.1 or D.2.2) if spit is green or yellow, (always ask
the victim to spit into a tissue and look at the color) or if there is
fever.

local anesthetic (D.17), preferably long-acting [bupivacaine]
injected directly into a rib fracture relieves pain for 24 hours, but
beware of slipping the needle between the ribs and puncturing the
lung.

Deep breathing exercises improve aeration of the lungs. In order
to clear secretions encourage coughing by holding the lower chest
for support. Inhale steam from a pot of boiling water in order to
liquefy junk in the chest and to make spit easier to cough up. Do
not splint the chest with strapping or bandages, which diminish
breathing movement and encourage pneumonia.

MECHANISM OF CHEST INJURY
The chest is a bony cage that acts like a bellows; it expands as the ribs
move upwards and outwards, and as the diaphragm moves downwards
like a piston. Quiet breathing, done by the diaphragm alone, is seen as
a gentle rise and fall of the upper abdomen with just a little movement
of the chest. Deep or labored breathing uses the intercostal muscles
between the ribs and accessory muscles in the neck. The lungs are
suspended inside the chest cavity, which together with the lung surface
are covered by pleura, a membrane that allows the two surfaces to slide
over each other without friction. The lung is normally held expanded
against the chest wall by a vacuum in the pleural space which, if
destroyed, causes the lung to collapse (pneumothorax). The air passages
branch like a tree: trachea, bronchi, bronchioles and alveoli, finally the
terminal air sacs.

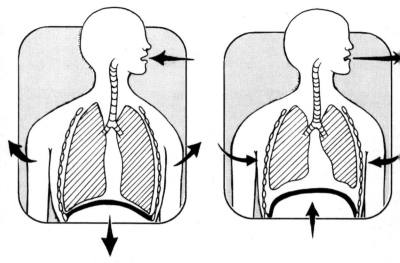

Mechanics of breathing

Look, feel, listen

Look at the victim in good light. He may show few signs of injury; his color will be difficult to see if he is unwashed and weather-beaten or if seen inside a colored tent. Open his clothing to display the whole chest, not just inside the top shirt button. Bluish lips (cyanosis) indicate inadequately oxygenated blood. Shock pales the face and accentuates cyanosis, present anyway in most climbers above 4,000m (13,000ft). Blood-flecked spittle suggests lung edema. A skin wound or bruising of the chest points to the injured side. After injury breathing is shallow, irregular, rapid (more than 30 breaths/minute), and the chest moves less on the injured side. Breathing and coughing are painful. When breathing is severely stressed the nostrils flare, neck muscles are taut and intercostal muscles are indrawn.

Feel the rib cage gently for tenderness and for an unstable

segment of chest wall. Place your palms flat on the sides of his bare chest; they should move apart equally with each breath. Crackling of air bubbles in the tissues (surgical emphysema) feels like paper being rustled.

Listen for the croaking sound of obstructed breathing and for a hiss of air escaping from, or the sucking noise of air entering, a chest wound.

Chest wall injury

SIMPLE RIB FRACTURES
Fractured ribs are usually caused by a direct blow. The resulting bruise can hide a liter of blood. Ribs can fracture spontaneously after a violent bout of coughing at high altitude. Severe pain, especially on breathing, comes from broken rib ends grating against sensitive overlying periosteum. Tenderness is felt over the point of fracture. Fractured ribs heal on their own in 3 to 6 weeks but remain painful during most of that time especially on deep breathing. Pain leads to shallow breathing and discourages coughing so secretions accumulate and become infected. Yellow or green spit, perhaps with blood, indicates pneumonia — the dreaded complication of chest injury.

MULTIPLE RIB FRACTURES
When several ribs are fractured and the chest wall is pushed in, jagged rib ends may puncture the underlying lung releasing air into the pleura (pneumothorax) or tear the intercostal vessels causing blood to pool in the chest (hemothorax). It is impossible to differentiate between these two in the outdoors; you may notice the lung on one side is collapsed, but to tell which side is not easy (see below).

Fractures of ribs 9, 10 and 11 on the left side may damage the spleen, on the right side the liver. If the pleural lining of the chest wall is breached air may leak into the tissues (surgical emphysema) and creep up into the neck where bubbles are felt crackling under the skin.

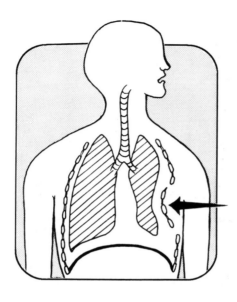

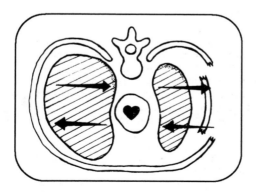

Flail chest

FLAIL CHEST

If several ribs are broken in two places a segment of chest wall is isolated like an island and moves in the opposite direction to the rest of the chest during breathing. It is sucked in on inspiration when the chest normally expands and is blown out on expiration when the chest deflates (paradoxical breathing). All the effort of breathing is spent in moving the unsupported flail segment rather than shifting air into and out of the lungs, which become poorly ventilated causing the victim to become cyanosed and go blue from lack of oxygen. Extra effort to breathe increases the paradoxical movement making the situation worse, so he becomes anxious, restless and sweaty.

Act: mild paradoxical breathing may need no treatment. If severe enough to cause distress fix the mobile segment of chest wall by pressing on it. The victim will immediately breathe more easily and become pink again. Tape a wound dressing over the injured ribs and turn him on that side in order to splint the broken ribs under the weight of his own body and prevent the segment of chest wall moving in and out.

If this fails endotracheal intubation or cricothyrotomy and artificial ventilation may be necessary along with rapid evacuation to a hospital.

Lung injury

PNEUMOTHORAX OR HEMOTHORAX

Air or blood can enter the pleural space either from outside by way of a penetrating wound, or from within due to an alveolus ruptured by a fractured rib, or spontaneously in a healthy young person. The vacuum in the pleural space is then destroyed so the lung, or part of it, collapses. Air sealed in the chest may be absorbed slowly and the lung will re-expand; if not, air may have to be drawn off through a needle.

To decide which lung is collapsed may be very difficult even with a stethoscope; it is vital to be sure because needling the one good lung might collapse it. With the victim breathing through his mouth listen carefully for breath sounds, which will be decreased or absent on the affected side. If breathing becomes restricted by a collapsed lung and the victim looks as if he will die, decompress the chest with a needle.

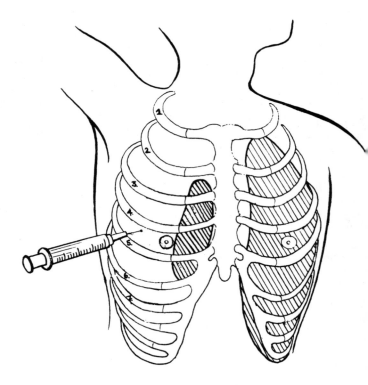

Pneumothorax, needling

Act: push a wide-bore needle between the ribs at or above the level of
the nipple in a line vertically below the mid-point of the axilla between
the folds that make the armpit. Point the needle upwards and
backwards to where a chest tube would be placed if such were
practicable. Allow a hiss of air to escape as he breathes out, then seal
the needle with a finger when he breathes in. When all the air appears
to have escaped, or blood has been sucked off, pull out the needle and
cover the hole with tape. A simple one-way valve can be made by tying

a condom tightly onto the needle and cutting off the rubber tip.
Decompression may have to be repeated if the chest fills up again.
Underwater seal drainage is preferable for continuous decompression in
hospital.

TENSION PNEUMOTHORAX
Urgent, on-the-spot, definitive action is needed, because tension
pneumothorax kills fast, especially at altitude. If a lung wound does not
seal on its own a flap of tissue may act as a one-way valve, so air is
sucked in with each breath but the flap-valve is closed on expiration.
This causes pressure on the mediastinum (trachea, heart and great
vessels) and obstructs return of blood to the heart, and also its output.
Air can be removed with a needle as described above. A simple
pneumothorax will not kill, but a tension pneumothorax may.

8 SHOCK

Shock is a vague term that describes how the body reacts to life under threat when the effective circulating blood volume is suddenly reduced. Shock may be caused by severe hemorrhage, major burns, profuse vomiting and diarrhea, overwhelming infection, acute pain or emotion and heart failure.

> In hemorrhagic shock a chain reaction unfolds. Bleeding reduces the volume of blood returning to the heart, which consequently pumps less blood into the circulation. The fall in blood pressure is sensed by receptors in the carotid arteries which cause the heart to speed up and to push out more blood in an attempt to keep the brain and vital organs adequately oxygenated. In order to pool blood in the center of the body blood vessels in the extremities of the limbs and the gut clamp down; the skin is by-passed and turns cold, pale and waxy-blue like death.
>
> If shock is not reversed the victim becomes breathless, thirsty and sick; finally he is restless and confused. Unless blood pressure is restored to normal by blood transfusion or intravenous fluids he will fall unconscious and may die. Prolonged low blood pressure causes irreversible changes in kidneys, adrenals, heart and brain. If left too late he may die even if blood is replaced.

Once severe bleeding is staunched write a record of the victim's progress as a baseline to assess whether he is improving or worsening. With hidden bleeding these observations may be the only guide to his condition.

Symptoms and signs of shock

Rapid, feeble pulse: over 120/minute. The force of the pulse against the examining fingers is only a rough guide to blood pressure, which requires a sphygmomanometer for accurate measurement.

Pale, cold, clammy, bluish skin: normal skin is pink and warm.

Capillary blood flow: the big toe-nail or thumb-nail blanches when squeezed, the normal pink color returning instantly on release of pressure; the speed of return is a good indicator of general blood pressure. Delay of several seconds, with cold hands and feet, and a cold nose, suggests shock or dehydration.

Restless behaviour: especially true of children in shock.

Thirst: unquenchable.

Dry, furred tongue: usually becomes moist again after two or three days when the ability to eat and drink returns. Encourage drinking fruit juice to restore lost potassium.

Low urine output: collect and measure all urine over a 12 hour period, in dehydration it is dark and concentrated. A normal person passes more than 25ml of pale and dilute urine each hour, indicating that fluid intake is adequate.

Sluggish gut movement: shock can paralyse the intestines and the victim may vomit. His gut does not absorb water adequately and his belly may become distended (paralytic ileus).

VISIBLE BLOOD LOSS
Estimating blood loss in soaked garments is often misleading but it indicates roughly the gravity of the injury and how much blood needs replacing. An egg-cupful of blood on a white shirt looks like an ocean to a lay observer, who is more likely to exaggerate than to underestimate blood loss. An injury may appear minor on the front of the victim but a liter or more may have soaked into the clothing and sleeping bag he is lying on.

INVISIBLE BLOOD LOSS
In closed wounds blood spreads along tissue planes causing swelling, or into body cavities displacing and irritating the contents. The available space dictates the direction and pressure of the swelling. A fractured femur can bleed a liter into the thigh making it swell to twice normal girth; the swelling may extend up to the hip and down to the knee.

  Act: Fluid replacement: if the victim feels thirsty give sips of water enough to quench thirst without making him vomit. After bleeding body water is drawn into the blood by osmotic pressure in order to compensate for lost plasma. Although not as good as replacing blood intravenously, fluid by mouth goes some way in helping to redress the upset body water balance.

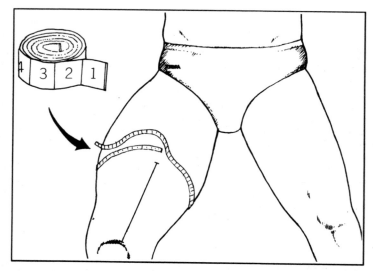

Blood-loss in fractured femur

The best composition for oral rehydration is the WHO formula (D.18).

Blood lost should be replaced ideally with blood, but this is rarely possible outside hospital. Other intravenous fluids (normal saline or Ringer's lactate), if brought by the rescuers, should be started before evacuating the victim in order to swell his plasma volume and alleviate shock. An intravenous drip provides a route for administering drugs in finely controlled doses.

Position: keep the victim's body tilted head down so blood will flow by gravity to the brain and prevent shock and loss of consciousness. With head wounds keep the head up.

Raise the feet above the level of the heart by placing them on a rucksack. About 2 liters of blood, pooled in the legs, is thereby returned to the central circulation. Elevate the wounded part because gravity lowers the pressure in arteries and veins locally and allows clotting.

COMFORT

Rest slows the heart while exercise speeds it. Resting the injured part encourages clotting and prevents a delicate web of early clot being broken or dislodged. Having dressed, packed, and bandaged the wound, splint it like a fracture and leave it undisturbed.

Pain makes a person restless even if unconscious. Half-measures are useless; treat severe pain in a fit adult with full doses of morphine (D.1.4) provided there is no breathing difficulty or head injury when codeine (D.1.3) is the drug of choice. Most chest injury victims breathe better when pain is relieved. As well as easing pain, these drugs give a pleasant feeling of warmth and well-being.

Reassure the victim that bleeding is under control because, humane considerations apart, anxiety quickens the pulse and raises the blood pressure. Warmth is akin to comfort. Clothe the victim and shelter him from the elements. He will probably feel cold because of some degree of shock.

Appearance of other sorts of bleeding

The commonest cause of bleeding is from wounds, but in wilderness you should be aware of other sorts of bleeding and the varied appearance of spilled blood. For more detail on the conditions mentioned here refer to appropriate chapters later in this book.

SALIVA

A nosebleed, bitten tongue, bleeding gums or tooth socket, injury to the nose, mouth or pharynx may cause bright red blood to trickle into the throat. It may be spat out mixed with saliva either as streaks or lumps of clot, or it may be swallowed. Look carefully with a strong light for the source of bleeding. One very serious cause is by a fracture of the base of the skull, when blood may also come from the ears, but in both cases it is mixed with watery cerebro-spinal fluid.

SPUTUM

Pink flecks coughed up in frothy phlegm suggest blood from the lungs, possibly due to pneumonia, pulmonary edema or embolus (fluid or clot in the lungs).

VOMIT

Swallowed blood irritates the stomach causing vomiting. If blood has lain for more than a day in the stomach it becomes partly digested and changes color from bright red to dark brown like coffee grounds. Having excluded the causes above, a bleeding peptic ulcer is most likely.

URINE

Scanty blood turns the urine cloudy or slightly orange; if profuse, a deep wine-red color. If peeing causes burning pain look for infection. When the story tells of a blow in the flank, suspect bleeding from the kidney. If pain is acute, colicky, and extremely severe, a stone in the urinary passages is possible.

STOOL

A little bright-red blood streaked on the toilet paper suggests a crack at the anal margin caused by a small pile (hemorrhoid), or by passing a constipated stool. Piles can bleed alarmingly, with clots. Digested blood (from an ulcer) that has passed the length of the gut produces, 6 to 8 hours later, a dark or tarry stool which can be confused with the black stool of someone taking iron tablets or an over-the-counter indigestion medication [Pepto-Bismol].

VAGINA

Normal menstrual rhythms are often interrupted by an energetic style of living, particularly on wilderness trips. The history of a missed period suggests pregnancy, so consider the diagnosis of a miscarriage (abortion) or a ruptured ectopic pregnancy in someone with vaginal bleeding.

9 LIMB INJURY

Soft tissue injuries

Injury to muscles, tendons, and ligaments are common in wilderness but are important, far exceeding their severity, because they hamper the escape of an injured person to safety.

BRUISES AND CONTUSIONS
Muscle hematoma — A muscle blood vessel broken by a blunt blow, for example in the thigh or buttock, can leak a liter of blood into surrounding soft tissues. This forms a tense, painful swelling (hematoma) which may take weeks to subside.
   Act: if the swelling has a soft center plunge a wide-bore needle into it after carefully cleaning the skin. If you strike gold, a fluid of that color will flow out; this is serum from broken down blood cells.

Subperiosteal hematoma — A blow on a bone near the skin surface, for example on the front of the shin, may cause bleeding under the periosteum, the thin membrane that enwraps bone and under which run nerves and blood vessels. The pooled blood-bruise lifts the periosteum, stretching it and causing much pain and tenderness. But the volume of blood that collects is less than in loose muscle tissue because the tension that builds also compresses the bleeding vessels. So subperiosteal hematomas rarely need to be drained.
   Act: rest, elevation and ice quell further bleeding and reduce swelling.

SPRAINS AND STRAINS
Ligaments and muscles may be stretched or torn when a joint is bent beyond its normal range of movement, yet the bones remain intact. A sprain swells immediately, usually round a joint; it hurts and is very tender. A sprain is not deformed, which distinguishes it from a displaced fracture or a dislocation. If the joint can be stressed by bending it past its normal limits, a ligament tear is

likely. A severe sprain is as crippling as a fracture, and can take as long, or longer, to heal. Ankles, knees, and thumbs are commonly sprained by outdoorsmen.

Act: cool the part with ice, snow or stream water for 15 minutes in each hour to reduce swelling and relieve pain. Rest the elevated limb above the level of the body in order to reduce bleeding and swelling. Support the joint firmly with tape or elastic bandage.

TEARS
Commonly torn are knee and ankle ligaments, Achilles and biceps tendons, and knee cartilages.

Act: immobilize tears by splinting; surgical correction can follow later.

TENDONITIS, BURSITIS, ARTHRITIS
Inflammation of a tendon, bursa (a fluid-filled cushion beneath a tendon) or a joint is painful and incapacitating because the underlying joint becomes stiff. Examples are shoulder (subacromial bursitis), elbow (epicondylitis), hip (trochanteric bursitis) and heel (Achilles tendonitis).

Act: rest, elevate, ice.

Rx: paracetamol (D.1.1) relieves pain and naproxen (D.1.2) reduces inflammation.

VEINS
Rupture, from blunt injury will cause a big hematoma (e.g. long saphenous vein). Inflammation causes thrombo-phlebitis.

SUPERFICIAL THROMBO-PHLEBITIS
The vein becomes tender, hardened into a cord, and the overlying skin turns red (e.g. varicose veins of the leg; forearm veins after i/v injection).

DEEP THROMBO-PHLEBITIS
Deep veins of the legs can become inflamed and clot (thrombosis) particularly if a climber lies around storm-bound at altitude and does not drink enough. The blood then becomes viscous, treacly and liable to clot forming a pulmonary embolus — a very serious matter (see below). Pain arises deep in the calf; feet and ankles

swell. Pushing on the ball of the foot to bring the big toe nearer the knee-cap causes pain deep in the calf (Homan's sign). The temperature is raised.

Act: rest with legs elevated and bandaged from groin to ankle until at least 3 days after all pain has subsided. Then evacuate urgently.

PULMONARY EMBOLUS

When a clot from a deep vein thrombosis in the calf detaches, the resulting embolus travels to, and through, the heart coming to rest in the lungs. A big clot can kill owing to massive right heart failure; in a less severe case the victim is shocked, breathless, and cyanosed. Sudden pain in the chest may be confused with heart attack. Cough produces blood-stained, often frothy, sputum. Deep breathing hurts.

Cerebral embolus — A "stroke" causes one side of the face or the body to become weak or paralysed.

Bony injuries

JOINT DISLOCATION

Dislocation occurs when one bone in a joint is displaced. The signs are similar to a fracture — swelling, deformity, pain, loss of use — but the diagnosis is usually obvious from the abnormal position of the joint compared with its uninjured opposite.

Act: attempt to reduce a dislocation in the same way as a fracture. If done immediately it may be quite easy, but after a few minutes the muscles overlying the joint go into tight spasm and nothing short of a general anesthetic will relax them. Nerves and blood vessels lie close to joints so always feel for pulses before trying to reduce a dislocation. Surrounding ligaments and soft tissues may be torn. Do not be deterred from having the courage to try to reduce a dislocation that may help a crippled person to help himself and others retreat safely.

Rx: morphine (D.1.4); then pull firmly and steadily (traction) in the axis of the limb with an assistant giving counter-traction in the opposite direction, before attempting any specific maneuver to reduce the dislocation (see specific dislocations p. 101).

FRACTURE

To fracture is to break, no more no less; but a fractured femur
sounds more dramatic than a broken thigh. Just as a chair-leg will
break if you knock, bend, twist, pull or crush it beyond certain
limits, so will bones break or crack. The difference is that wood is
inert but bone is a plastic, living framework wrapped in a tough
membrane of periosteum to which muscles, tendons and ligaments
are attached. Periosteum is rich in nerve fibers and registers most
of the pain of a broken bone. Bones mend in the same way as
wounds heal.

   The distinction between closed and open fractures is important
in practical care. A closed fracture has intact overlying skin that
is breached in an open fracture. Whether skin is broken from
within by jagged bone ends, or by force from outside, the
underlying fractured bone is open to infection, which delays
healing, smoulders and may progress to deep infection of bone
(osteomyelitis) — a dreaded complication.

   All fractures need splinting to prevent the broken fragments
moving against each other and causing pain and further damage
to neighboring muscles, nerves and blood vessels. Stable fractures,
which are immoble, may become unstable if inadequately
supported.

EXAM

Ask how the accident happened, whether the victim heard the
crack of breaking bone, where he feels pain, and whether he can
move the part himself.

   Look at the limb. Remove clothing, if necessary by cutting
along seams. Always compare the injured side with its uninjured
normal opposite side; slight swelling or deformity become obvious
at a glance.

   Feel the limb beginning away from the area of pain and
gradually working towards it. Watch the victim's face constantly;
nothing will be learned from staring at your examining hands,
whereas even a flicker of pain will register on his face. Hurting a
person is inexcusable and many medical students have failed their
final exams for doing so.

Shock (in fractures) — The victim may be emotionally shocked
because of severe pain or anxiety about the outcome of the

accident, a forced bivouac or a rescue call-out. He may also be in physiological shock from loss of blood into the tissues causing a lowered blood volume with low blood pressure and rapid pulse. A severely fractured femur may cause a liter of blood to collect in soft tissues around the bone (i.e. 1/5 of the total blood volume). Bleeding comes from the bone marrow cavity, vessels in the periosteum and surrounding muscle, and tissues torn by the jagged bone ends. With multiple fractures and open wounds the blood loss may be fatal.

Signs and symptoms of fractures

Pain — Most fractures cause a dull ache; when the bone fragments move suddenly causing the ends to grate, or the periosteum to stretch, they become excruciatingly painful. Tenderness is invariable, and gentle pressure over even a small break causes pain, which worsens shock.

Swelling — Hidden bleeding and edema fluid cause swelling, which can be reduced by rest, elevation and ice. Bruising appears later as blood seeps through to the skin.

Open wounds need special care before splinting in order to avoid infection. Clear away dirt and debris, and wash the wound with copious water and soap; cover with a bulky sterile dressing held firmly in place with tape.

Rx: broad-spectrum antibiotic (D.2) and tetanus toxoid as soon as possible.

Deformity — Correcting a severe angular deformity early, before swelling and muscle spasm develop, is safe and harmless provided it can be done without undue resistance from, or pain to, the victim. Go ahead:

— if you have the expertise and confidence to do so, knowing it will take many days to reach help;
— if the bone is markedly mal-aligned and in peril of stretching or pinching nerves or blood vessels (check for the return of an absent pulse after straightening);
— if the skin is taut and blanched, suggesting the blood supply is compromised by pressure from within.

Loss of use — The victim will hold the part quite still, guarding it from pain. Let him do so; this is Nature's splinting. Loss of use strongly suggests fracture, because pain and instability discourage movement.

Associated damage — Damage to soft tissues around the fracture may be worse than the bone injury itself:

— blood vessels tear and bleed. Pinching an artery in the fracture, or spasm resulting from irritation by a broken bone, restricts circulation to the whole limb. Tissues around a fracture swell and hamper blood flow.
— skin is weakened by swelling, stretching and bruising. Broken skin changes a closed fracture into an open one. Blood flow is usually adequate if the skin beyond the injury is warm and pink. Beware if skin goes blue or white, remains blanched on pressure, and if the pulse is absent.
— nerves may be damaged causing numbness, loss of pain and sensation, and paralysis.

Act: if the person is only severely bruised or suffering a sprain he may, after firm taping, be able to continue unaided. If a leg is fractured he will have to be carried or assisted, with added delay and danger. With a suspected fracture loosen tight clothing and avoid bandages that restrict circulation. Splinting is the key to managing fractures because, once an unstable bone is immobilized, the victim can be handled with less pain and further damage is avoided. Complete immobilization is possible only in a plaster cast.

Reducing a fracture — Before trying to reduce a fracture reassure the victim and quietly explain what you intend to do so he will be as relaxed as possible, and not be surprised by sudden movement.

Rx: morphine (D.1.4); a nip of brandy will relax the victim, but alcohol is not a pain-killer.

Exert traction, best done with two people pulling in opposite directions. Take a firm grasp on uninjured skin well away from the fracture and gently pull on the limb for 3 to 5 minutes to overcome muscle spasm; a helper holds the limb near the trunk, giving counter-traction. Handle the limb in one piece so the bone-

ends do not grate. Sudden painful movement will cause the
overlying muscles to lock firmly in spasm; any chance of reducing
the fracture, especially in a muscular victim, will be slight.
Traction usually removes pain; if it persists keep pulling before
attempting to reduce the fracture. It also improves circulation and
nerve function across the fracture site.

Reduce the fracture by increasing traction gently, firmly,
resolutely and without hurry. Watch the victim's face all the time
to ensure he is not being hurt unnecessarily. Once the bone ends
are separated pain is relieved and it is easier to restore them to
their natural position ready for splinting. But do not relax traction
until the limb is splinted. Do not persist in hurting the victim by
seeking perfect alignment. Aim to get the bone roughly straight;
an orthopedic surgeon can tidy up any angulation problems later.

Splinting — Splint a fracture so the joint above and below the
break are immobile. Splinting may be delayed if being trussed up
in an awkward situation means the victim cannot help in his own
evacuation to a safer place. If he has to be carried on a stretcher,
pad below weight-bearing points (e.g. heels) and between bony
prominences (e.g. ankles) using spare clothing or a ring-pad like a
dough-nut. Fill hollows under the knees. Tie splinting bandages
firmly but not so tight as to impede circulation. Leave toes and
fingers open to view so their color and temperature can be
observed; undo the whole splint and bandage if they become pale,
blue or cold. With swelling a tight splint can quickly become a
tourniquet. Wilderness guides should practice making splints
before a trip; when improvising a splint in earnest try it on the
uninjured limb first.

Body Splints: The most available splint is the body itself. A
broken arm can be splinted to the chest and a broken leg to the
opposite uninjured leg with padding in between.

Improvised Splints: Imagination designs improvised splints;
surgical tape will secure them in place.
— Arm: closed-cell foam pad, cut to size; bark peeled from
    birch, poplar, alder or any hardwood; newspaper or a
    magazine rolled into a tube; cardboard cut and shaped to an
    angled gutter.

— Leg: tree branch or ice axe; tent pole, ice picket, ski, telescopic ski pole, canoe paddle.

— Ankle: down jacket, clothing.

— Back: two pack-frames strapped together; a cabin door or a ladder; 2 paddles.

— Crutch: trim a stout sapling at a Y-junction.

Malleable Splints: Kramer wire; wire mesh ¼″. Bend to conform to the shape needed.

Inflatable Splints (often carried by rescue teams): The limb is put into an inflatable double-skinned tube, different sizes for arms and legs. Leg splints wrap around the limb and are closed by a zip-fastener or Velcro self-adhesive material. Put an arm splint over your own arm, wrist-end first. Grasp the victim's hand, as in greeting, and slide the splint from your arm onto his. Inflatable splints can be blown up too tight and cut off blood supply; no harm will come if they are inflated by mouth so they can still be easily indented with finger pressure. They must be let down every 2 hours and re-inflated. Always leave the fingers and toes open for inspection of color and temperature. Inflatable splints fold away neatly and can be put on over clothing. With careful handling they should not puncture. If evacuating the person by air, splints must be partially deflated because of pressure change at altitude.

Plaster Splints: Fibreglass (C-cast) should replace Plaster of Paris for wilderness rescue because it is light, waterproof and durable, though expensive. It makes a rigid cast that can be moulded to the limb. A back-slab is the safest plaster splint for an arm or leg. The cast is moulded onto the natural contour of the back of the limb encasing not more than ¾ of the circumference so the remaining gap allows the limb to expand if it swells. The limb is wrapped in a light bandage, shirt or under-clothes; and the plaster is put on over it. The limb should be on slight traction in the normal position at rest. Don't aim at perfect position as the cast can be replaced on reaching hospital.

Never apply plaster directly to the skin; put it on over padding either of wool or the victim's clothing left in place. Fold any loose ends back so the skin does not rub when the plaster hardens. Wear a pair of large disposable surgical gloves to apply the plaster; they should be packed with the rolls in the medical kit.

Traction splints: useful for lower limb fractures. The Thomas splint has been used for over a century (see p. 112). It is still useful for rescue teams but is too bulky and heavy to be carried even by a small expedition. In order to give the same effect a traction device can be improvised from two pack-frames lashed together, or two ski poles.

Specific injuries

The common bony injuries in wilderness accidents are to the spine, pelvis, ribs, collar-bone, forearm, hand, lower leg, and ankle. For convenience, specific injuries will be dealt with region by region.

Upper limb

Injuries around the shoulder, collar-bone (clavicle), upper arm (humerus), elbow or forearm (radius and ulna) can be immobilized with a sling and swathe to bind the limb to the chest. The weight of the arm itself gives some traction for upper arm injuries. A forearm sling is easily made with a triangular bandage or a collar-and-cuff. The sleeve of the victim's jacket can be pinned to his opposite shoulder. A swathe of rope or clothing, padded for comfort, binds and splints the injured arm to the chest.

CLAVICLE
Fractured clavicle: the clavicle lies close under the skin so any break in normal contour is easily seen.

Act: a forearm sling and swathe is preferable for a day or two, but if pain persists a figure-of-8 bandage will brace the shoulders back and prevent the broken bone-ends grating. Leave the jacket on and make two well-padded rings, one for each shoulder, out of bandage or a scarf. Use a third tie to windlass the rings together and pull the shoulders back; pad between this cross-piece and the spine. If the hands tingle or go numb, slacken the windlass.

Acromio-clavicular joint separation: the tip of the shoulder is very tender and hurts to move. A high step in the contour is obvious.

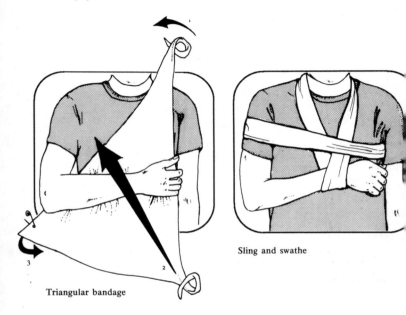

Triangular bandage

Sling and swathe

Act: a sling makes the joint comfortable until it heals, but accurate reduction is unnecessary unless very widely separated; then a surgeon is needed.

SHOULDER
Shoulder dislocation: A fairly common and dramatic injury whereby the head of the humerus, that forms the upper arm, slips below the shallow socket (glenoid) of the shoulder blade (scapula) in which it lies. With prompt attention a person, disabled and in pain, can be enabled to assist in his own evacuation. Every first-aider should learn how to reduce and replace a shoulder dislocation because it is one of the few medical emergencies where swift, skilful intervention by a layman can make a significant difference to the outcome. The procedure is satisfying to victim and rescuer alike, hence the space devoted to it here.

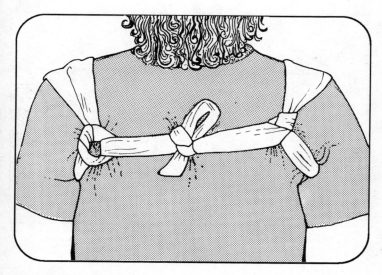

Figure-of-eight bandage

A first-time dislocation, usually from a fall on an outstretched hand, needs to be reduced within minutes or else the powerful muscles around the shoulder go into spasm and lock tight because of pain. Recurrent dislocation of the shoulder affects some people, but the shoulder is easily replaced, often under the instruction of the victim himself.

EXAM

Look: the rounded contour of the shoulder is lost, compared with the normal side, and the shoulder tip is pointed and angulated with the upper arm lying away from the chest. The victim supports his injured arm with the opposite hand.

Act: reassure the victim and help him to relax his shoulder muscles with gentle massage. Before attempting to reduce a dislocated shoulder feel for a radial pulse and test for sensation of

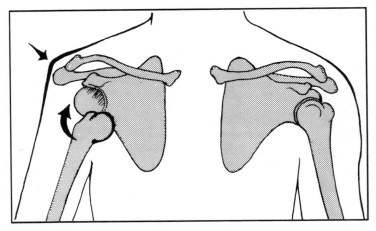

Dislocated shoulder

touch. Record any abnormal findings because nerves and blood vessels may get pinched in the armpit (axilla), especially if there is an associated fracture of the neck of the humerus. A pinched circumflex nerve, the commonest injury, causes an area of loss of feeling over the outer upper arm 5cm below the tip of the shoulder.

Rx: morphine (D.1.4) before attempting reduction.

Lie the victim face down for 15 to 30 mins with the injured arm hanging over the side of the elevated surface where he is lying. Tie a weight, like a pack-sack, to the wrist of the injured side in order to give extra traction; this alone may reduce the shoulder. If it does not, turn the victim over, have an assistant pull the arm gently to 90° from the body. Then push up with both thumbs on the head of the humerus which can be felt in the armpit.

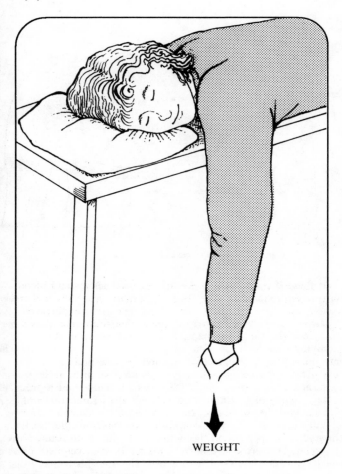

WEIGHT

Reducing dislocated shoulder

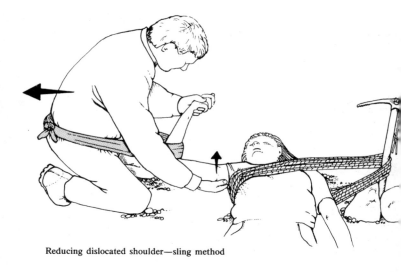

Reducing dislocated shoulder—sling method

If these simple measures fail try the *Two-sling* or the
Hippocrates method:

Two-sling: is least likely to cause further damage but requires
practice. The slings can be made of rolled cloth, a belt, a
climbing sling, or rope. One sling, well-padded, passes under the
armpit of the victim's dislocated shoulder and pulls across the
body (counter-traction) either towards an assistant kneeling
opposite, or to a fixed point like a tree, a boulder, or a piton in
place. Gently move the injured arm 90° away from the trunk
(abduction); bend, or flex, the elbow to 90°.

Put the other sling first round the crook of the elbow of the
injured arm, then round the buttocks of you, the rescuer. Kneel,
or squat, beside the victim. With your left hand keep 90° of elbow
flexion on the victim's arm, raised to 90° from his trunk. Place
your right hand in his arm-pit feeling for the head of the
humerus. Lean back into the loop sling in order to give a strong,
steady pull on the victim's arm. Rotate his arm slightly using his
forearm to lever the head of the humerus gently over the lip of the

shoulder joint rim (glenoid), while pushing lightly with your right hand on the head of the humerus. It should go in with a satisfying pop, and the victim's face will light up with joy.

Hippocrates: place your own socked foot as high in the victim's armpit as possible, hold his wrist with both hands and lean backwards with your knee and leg straight. Give a long and steady pull on his arm and push with your heel. This traction will ease his pain immediately. Talk to the victim reassuringly in order to get him to relax.

After at least 5 minutes traction, gear yourself up mentally for one strong, smooth movement to reduce the shoulder; if you fail the shoulder will go into spasm again and you have lost your chance. While maintaining your push-pull on his arm, lever his hand across his body using your heel as a fulcrum. The head of the humerus should slip back into the socket with a slight clunk.

Put the arm in a sling and bind it firmly to the chest. It should be X-rayed as soon as possible, ideally before effecting any of these maneuvers, in order to exclude a fracture, but this is obviously not possible in wilderness.

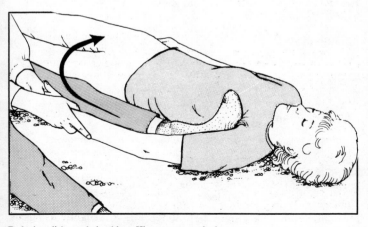

Reducing dislocated shoulder—Hippocrates method

Painful Shoulder (tendonitis, bursitis, frozen shoulder etc): many lesions around the shoulder result from bruising, injury or overuse. Movement is painful and limited.

Fracture of the humerus: reduction is unnecessary; use a full arm sling or a collar-and-cuff wrist sling leaving the elbow unsupported to give gravity traction.

Rx: naproxen (D.1.2) and rest.

ELBOW

Fractures and dislocations around the elbow: common in children and difficult to distinguish between the two, so treat as the same. They are especially serious because the brachial artery and nerves crossing the crook of the elbow may be damaged by the broken bone ends or in attempts to reduce the fracture, always difficult task.

Act: if the radial pulse at the wrist is absent always attempt reduction and hope blood flow may return. If absent, splint the arm as you find it and get to hospital fast.

Tennis Elbow (lateral epicondylitis): the knob on the outer side of the elbow is tender on lifting a pot, shaking hands or hammering, because the origin of the extensor muscles on the back of the forearm is inflamed.

Act: place 1″ tape right round the forearm 2″ below the knob in order to make a false origin for the extensor muscles. Avoid activities that hurt and be patient for 3 to 6 months.

FOREARM

Fracture of the radius and ulna: usually occur together.

Act: splint with a slab on the back of the forearm including the elbow and swathe to the body.

WRIST

Colles' fracture (further end of radius and ulna): the wrist has the shape of a dinner fork and needs reducing by a surgeon.

Act: splint the forearm with the wrist slightly cocked backed. Kramer wire can be moulded to the shape of the wrist.

"Sprains": often hide an underlying fracture or a ligament tear, which may be serious; so always have them X-rayed.

Scaphoid fracture of the palm: tender over the "snuffbox"
between the tendons of the extended thumb, seen when the thumb
is cocked up. It may be complicated when the nearer fragment of
bone loses its blood supply and dies (avascular necrosis) as seen
on X-ray.

Bennett's fracture (sprained thumb): a chip at the base of the
thumb metacarpal needs to be screwed into place by a surgeon.

Skier's (gamekeeper's) thumb: disrupted ulnar collateral ligament.
The thumb is unstable and the ligament must be repaired
surgically.

Tendonitis: the tendons of the wrist hurt and may creak on
moving, often as a result of overuse.
  Rx: naproxen (D.1.2), rest, ice, firm bandage

HAND
Fractures of the small bones of the hand: splint in a "boxing
glove" with a rolled-up sock placed in the palm of the hand and

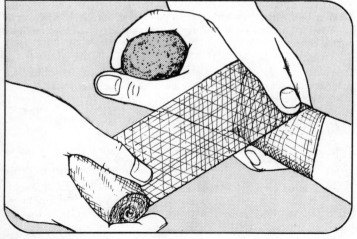

Boxing-glove dressing

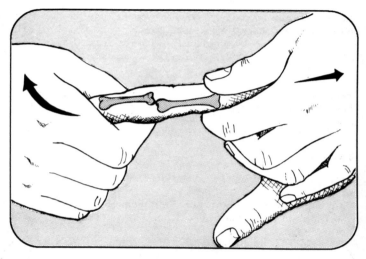

Reducing dislocated finger

make a bulky dressing with a tensor bandage leaving the fingers open for inspection — also a useful dressing for soft tissue injuries of the hand.

Dislocation of the finger or thumb: obvious from its deformity. A straight pull may not be effective because tissue becomes interposed between the ends. Flex the dislocated finger joint then pull while pushing the distal finger (or toe) back on. Splint the finger to its neighbor.

Tendon and nerve injuries: always serious; flexor tendons in the palm especially so. Surgery is urgent.

Infected hand or fingers: soak in hot water. If pus shows like a boil at the base of the nail (whitlow) or at the apex of the pulp (pulp abscess) first freeze it with ice, then knife it to drain the pus.
   Rx: antibiotic (D.2).

Slivers or splinters: cut a V-wedge over the sliver as far back as possible and try to grasp it with tweezers.

Sliced finger: replace and hold the flap with Steristrips. It may act as a graft and "take" with full healing.

Avulsion of a finger: keep the part in saline solution in a plastic bag. If a surgeon is reached quickly the piece may be able to be sewn on again.

Lower limb

HIP or THIGH
Fracture or dislocation of the head or neck of the femur: the difference may be difficult to tell but is important. In neither condition will the victim be able to walk and he will have much

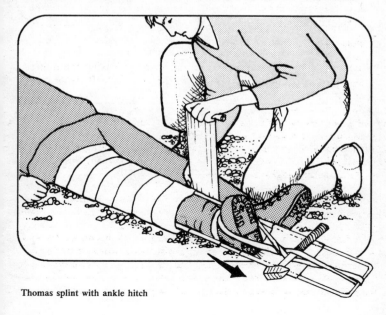

Thomas splint with ankle hitch

pain in the hip. A fracture is usually caused during a fall by landing on both feet; the hip is extended and rotated outwards. A dislocation is caused by a force directly on the knee bent at right angles; the hip is flexed and internally rotated and the femur is moved towards the mid-line and cannot be straightened. Massive contraction of the buttock and thigh muscles makes reduction extremely difficult.

Act (Fracture): a Thomas splint, or one of its modern derivatives can windlass the foot in order to pull the femur straight. Although unlikely to be available, the Thomas splint is described here in order to help you devise a way of rigging up a traction device from two pack-frames or other gear at hand.

> Thread the ring of the Thomas splint over the injured limb until it abuts against the pubic bone high up in the crotch. An assistant pulls on the victim's foot. The leg rests on supporting slings secured with safety pins between the arms of the splint. Tie an ankle-hitch over his boot with a bandage and secure it to the cross end-piece of the splint. Increase traction on the leg by windlassing the bandage, but beware not to overtighten it. If the victim complains of pain around the ankle-hitch slacken the tension. With his boot on you cannot see the color of his toes nor feel their temperature, so be aware of impeding the circulation.
>
> If you cannot make a traction device tie two ice-axes together to make a splint from armpit to ankle. Pad the picks well. Place binders round the whole body and bandage the bad leg to the good one with lots of padding between the legs.

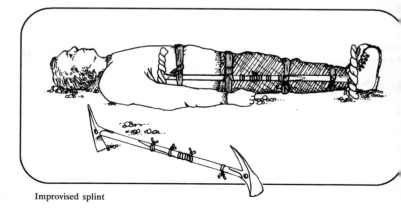

Improvised splint

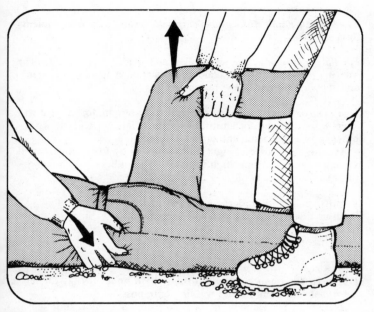

Reducing dislocated hip

Act (dislocation): with an assistant pressing down on the wings of the victim's pelvis, bend his knee to 90° and steady his foot between your knees, Give a long, strong pull upwards and gently rotate the hip. Reducing a hip without an anesthetic is almost impossible, but you may have to try if far from help. A Thomas splint is useless for reducing a hip, and anyway would be impossible to position owing to swelling.

Trochanteric bursitis: pain develops over the protuberance of the hip, and increases on walking.
    Rx: naproxen (D.1.2) and rest.

Ruptured saphenous vein: causes dramatic bruising and swelling, on the inside of the thigh, which will subside unaided.

KNEE

Knee fracture and dislocation: rare and results only from violent force.

Patella fracture: the knee is swollen and tender over the knee-cap where a dent may be felt. Patella dislocation is usually recurrent and the victim knows how to replace it.

Ligament or meniscus tears: difficult to differentiate; in both the knee is swollen and feels unstable. Pain is felt particularly when pressing over the joint line on the injured side.
   Act: hold the knee straight and immobile by firm support with a tensor bandage from thigh to ankle. The bulkier the dressing the steadier it will hold it.

Bursitis: pain and tenderness are felt in front of the patella (housemaids), below the patella (clergymen), or behind the hollow (climbers).
   Rx: naproxen (D.1.2) and rest.

LOWER LEG

Fractured tibia and/or fibula: usually both bones break, the leg is deformed and painful, and walking is impossible.
   Act: splint from above the knee to below the ankle and evacuate to a surgeon.

Ruptured gastrocnemius or Achilles tendon: the victim feels as though he has been booted in the mid-calf or above the heel. Walking is difficult and he cannot tip-toe.
   Act: the calf will heal on its own; the Achilles may need surgery.

Shin splints: embodies legion aches felt in the lower leg after over-use by hypochondriacal athletes. Rest is of the essence.

Thrombo-phlebitis: the calf is tender and flexing the foot towards the knee hurts in the calf. The danger is of a clot shooting to the lungs (embolus).
   Rx: analgesics (D.1), antibiotic (D.2) and rest until symptoms subside.

ANKLE

Sprains and fractures of the ankle: occur by tripping or falling
from a height. They are difficult to distinguish, especially a lateral
malleolus chip-fracture that is common in skiing and may be
diagnosed as a sprained or twisted ankle. Both are swollen and
painful. A fracture makes walking most unpleasant. If the heels
hurt suspect a fractured calcaneum and examine the spine as it
may also have been injured in the fall.

   Act: pillow-splint a fracture with a down jacket; splint a sprain
firmly with tape making a figure-of-8 around the ankle.

FOOT

Fractures of the small bones: occur when something heavy drops
on the foot, or after long marching — usually the 2nd metatarsal.
They are painful but not serious and can be strapped. The victim
should walk if possible; dallying may mean being benighted with
the peril that goes with an unplanned bivouac. To evacuate
someone by stretcher is slow, laborious and often dangerous. A
broken arm should not hinder progress, but a fractured leg will
probably be too painful to walk on and the victim will have to be
carried. Keep reviewing the condition of the person, and of his
limb, as you go. He may need a dressing loosened, a splint
adjusted, a pee, or another dose of pain-killer.

Ingrowing toe-nail: always cut toe-nails straight across to prevent a
sliver at the side digging in and becoming painfully infected.
   Act: warm salt soaks, cut a V-wedge in the middle of the nail.
   Rx: antibiotic (D.2).

Pelvis

FRACTURE

Falling from a height is the commonest cause of someone crushing
the ring of pelvic bones. The pelvis is surrounded by many
muscles and hollow spaces so a severe fracture may not be
obvious; the person's only complaint may be of pain round the
hips and difficulty in walking. Several pints of blood can seep into
the tissues unnoticed before he suddenly collapses from shock. He

may rupture his urethra or bladder as a result of the fractured pelvis (see p.128, ruptured urethra).

Act: pad the crotch with soft wool clothing and put a firm supporting binder round the upper thighs; bandage the knees and feet together to prevent the legs moving on the pelvis. Give analgesics and evacuate gently on a stretcher.

Belly

To distinguish one tender belly from another needs skill; ideally,
all of them need a surgeon. But until help can be reached use
intravenous fluids, antibiotics — and hope.

EXAM

Ask: where is the pain? (the areas where pain and tenderness
are felt usually overlie the organs; to describe the pain divide the
abdomen into quarters — right and left, upper and lower, flanks
to the side, loins behind). When and how did it start (exact time,
sudden or gradual)? Nature of pain (dull, aching, sharp, crampy)
and any change? Has pain moved? Does it radiate to another area
(to the back, shoulders, genitals)? Appetite loss, indigestion,
nausea, vomiting? Diarrhea, constipation? Peeing more frequent
or burning? Blood in the urine or stool?

Look: first at the victim's face. Is he well or ill, pale or flushed,
hot or cold, frowning in pain or calm and relaxed? Remove
clothing so you can see from chest to thigh. Scars of previous
surgery? Tongue moist or dry (as in dehydration or mouth-
breathing), clean or furred and smelly breath (as in appendicitis)?
Does the abdomen rise with normal breathing, is it held rigid with
the lower chest doing all the work, is it swollen or distended?
Local swelling, especially in the hernial areas?

Feel: the pulse, and temperature of the forehead using the back
of the fingers. Feel gently in all quarters of the belly with the flat
of a warm hand; don't dig with your fingers or he'll tense and you
will learn nothing. Does the abdomen let your hand sink in or
does it feel rigid, guarding the contents? Press in one spot; does it
hurt in another? Watch his face all the while for a grimace that
suggests tenderness. Only a large or solid mass will be palpable;
detecting a small mass requires much experience. Gently feel the
hernia areas in the groin, the scrotum and the testicles.

Listen: for normal gurgling bowel sounds with an ear placed
against his belly for at least 3 minutes; tinkling sounds tell that

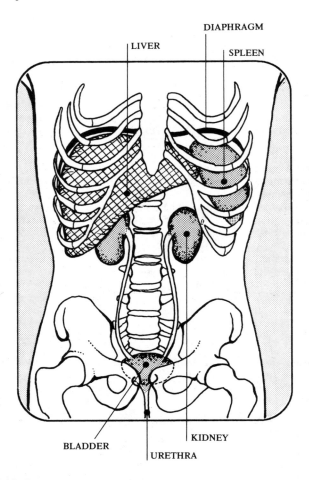

Abdominal organs

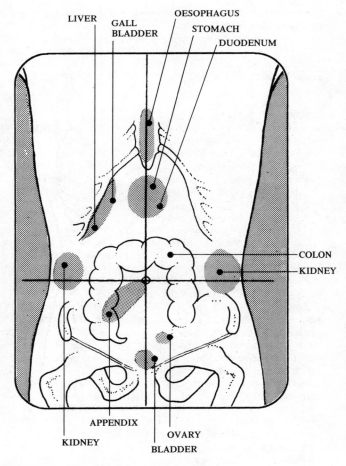

Areas (approximate) where abdominal organ pain is felt

the bowel is moving, silence suggests paralysis (ileus) possibly due to obstruction or peritonitis.

Draw a picture to record every finding.

Acute belly-ache can occur in the fit, young, and healthy. The most serious cause is appendicitis, which if neglected, can be deadly.

ACUTE APPENDICITIS
Appendicitis is easy to diagnose once all the classical signs are manifest, yet in its early stages it can be similar to several other conditions that cause abdominal pain. The finger-like appendix lies in the right lower quarter of the abdomen. Its variable position in relation to the large bowel, and its stage of inflammation, account for the variety of signs it presents.

Symptoms & Signs of appendicitis
Pain: commonly starts around the umbilicus and after about 6 hours shifts to the right lower quarter. The victim feels queasy, the idea of food is revolting, and he passes up French fries. Vomiting usually occurs after the onset of central pain and before it moves to the right side. Walking hurts in the right groin and he prefers to lie still with legs drawn up.

Look: he is unwell and flushed with fever; if the appendix perforates the pain eases and he looks pale and shocked owing to peritonitis. The pulse races. The tongue is furred and the breath stinks. Ask about previous surgery; a scar suggests that the appendix has already been snatched, If it has gone heave a sigh of relief because the diagnosis will be easier.

Feel: muscles in the right lower quarter guard the tender contents of his belly, whereas the left side remains soft and empty. Pressing more deeply where it hurts and, once only, releasing the pressure suddenly, may evoke an "ouch!" (rebound tenderness). Bowel sounds are absent if peritonitis has spread.

Act: an inflamed appendix can burst within 24 to 36 hours spilling pus into the belly and causing peritonitis, which may kill. If a surgeon cannot be reached swiftly stop feeding the person by mouth because drinking will make him vomit. Give intravenous fluids.

"Drip-and-suck" should tide the victim over till surgery using an intravenous infusion of normal saline or Ringer's solution run at about 3 liters over 24 hours. Suck out hourly the contents of a naso-gastric tube passed through the nose (or mouth if not possible) into the stomach and taped in place.

Rx: double doses of broad-spectrum antibiotic, cephalosporin (D.2.1), i/v would be best but i/m or oral route would do. Be generous with pain-killers.

If the victim is not cured by this time-honored ship-board regime, he may develop a mass with the appendix walled off by omentum (the fat-laden membrane that hangs from the bowel). An abscess forms like a time-bomb wrapped in a protective coat for later dismantling by a surgeon. The worst scenario is when the appendix bursts spilling pus into the peritoneum (peritonitis);

Rx: metronidazole (D.2.3) added to both antibiotics cephalosporin (D.2.1) and co-trimaxazole (D.2.2) in double doses.

The following conditions mimic appendicitis and have to be excluded when faced with acute low belly-ache, but in every case a surgeon should be consulted as soon as possible because an accurate diagnosis is very difficult to make in the wilderness. The conditions are arranged roughly in order of frequency:

CONSTIPATION

Inadequate drinking, lack of fresh fruit, eating dehydrated food, and medication containing morphine or codeine cause constipation. Prove with a laxative suppository or an enema; like clearing a log jam, it's best approached from below. An impacted, rock-hard stool may be the result of dehydration and constipation owing to being storm-bound in a tent and not melting enough snow in order to drink. If the stool has to be removed, push a greased finger as high in the rectum as possible breaking the hard stool and withdrawing it in pieces. A soapy water enema helps to flush out the residue.

GASTRO-ENTERITIS

Crampy pain, profuse and watery diarrhea, and nausea and vomiting are usual. The story may be of eating strange food (oysters, or Tibetan tea) or of other members of the party being

similarly stricken. Giardiasis occurs where beavers live in the
water and in other wild regions.

Act: avoid eating, drink plenty; diarrhea will probably cease in
24-48 hours, but if not,

Rx: immodium (D.9.3) and metronidazole (D.2.3) against the
Giardia.

URINARY TRACT INFECTION
The victim, commonly female, pees frequently (every 15 to 30
minutes), and it feels like passing powdered glass. Murky, smelly
urine may be tinged with blood. Pain and tenderness are felt in
the flank (kidney infection, pyelitis), or above the pubis (bladder
infection, cystitis), which mimic an inflamed appendix in contact
with the ureter or bladder. Despite a high fever she shakes with
chills.

Act: fluids in plenty with baking soda added in order to make
the urine alkaline and less clement to acid-loving E. coli.

Rx: co-trimoxazole (D.2.1) broad-spectrum antibiotic.

STONE IN THE KIDNEY OR URETER
So long as a stone remains in the kidney only a dull ache is felt in
the loin. Agonizing colic ("the worst pain I've ever felt") occurs
when a small stone passes down the ureter connecting kidneys and
bladder. Small stones, like small dogs, make most noise. The
victim rolls around with steady pain, which starts in the loin and
moves towards the groin, and often into the genitals. Pain comes
in waves, builds to a crescendo with vomiting, and then dies down
leaving a dull ache. Urine is passed frequently and may be blood-
stained.

Act: drink plenty in order to flush out the stone, take strong
pain-killers, and meditate whilst waiting for the passing of the
stone.

ACUTE GALLBLADDER
Constant severe pain, felt high under the right ribs, travels
through to the back, to the bottom of the lower right shoulder
blade, or to the right shoulder tip. Fatty foods cause indigestion.
A low-slung gallbladder may give pain down to the right lower
quarter like appendicitis. However, it is more likely to be confused

with a peptic ulcer or an inflamed esophagus. Yellow jaundice suggests a stone is obstructing the flow of bile, causing pale stools and dark urine.

Act: most attacks subside without surgery, so rest and give limited fluids.

Rx: codeine (D.1.3), (not morphine which constricts the bile-duct exit), and antibiotics (D.2).

WOMEN'S PROBLEMS
Pain from the right ovary or right fallopian tube can mimic appendicitis.

Ovary pain: Ask any woman complaining of low belly-ache the date of her last period, and whether she could be pregnant. The pain may be just her normal pre-menstrual pains which are sometimes quite disabling. If the date is exactly half-way between her periods she may be ovulating normally. Acute pain and tenderness lingering for a few hours may be due to slight bleeding from the ovarian follicle into the peritoneum (mittelschmertz).

Salpingitis: Infection of the fallopian tubes is usually accompanied by smelly vaginal discharge. Fever is high and pain is felt on both sides low down, but it may be over the appendix only.

If she is pregnant beware of:

Abortion (miscarriage): The story is of a missed period, heavy vaginal bleeding, and generalized cramps with passing of clots.
Rx: [ergometrine] 0.25 mg.i/m.

Ectopic pregnancy: Pregnancy develops on rare occasions outside the womb in one or other fallopian tube, which can suddenly burst causing profuse bleeding into the belly.
Act: only surgery avails; i/v fluids may help meanwhile.

INTESTINAL OBSTRUCTION
Any part of the bowel, large or small, may become obstructed by a multitude of causes, mostly too academic to discuss here. But look for a scar from previous surgery suggesting adhesions, or a hernia that may have twisted.

The bowel may distend, strangulate, die and burst leading to fatal peritonitis. Any obstruction on the right side of the belly may simulate appendicitis. The features are of a sick-looking person with pain, vomiting, distension and absolute constipation.

Rx: pain-killers (D.1), and antibiotics, cephalosporin (D.2.1) and metronidazole (D.2.3). Drip-and-suck.

PEPTIC ULCER

Ulcers in the stomach or duodenum can exist for years without causing more than vague indigestion and discomfort in the pit of the stomach coming on 1 to 2 hours after eating. Avoid fried foods, coffee, alcohol and cigarettes but drink milk. An ulcer may bleed or perforate suddenly and catastrophically.

Rx: aluminium hydroxide (D.9.1), famotidine (D.9.2).

Bleeding: The victim feels faint and sweaty, vomits bright-red or coffee-ground blood (hematemesis) and becomes shocked. Diarrhea may follow some hours later with dark, tarry stools (melena).

Act: drip-and-suck until it is possible to replace blood with blood

Rx: famotidine (D.9.2).

Perforation: Sudden pain in the upper abdomen can mimic a heart attack or a perforated appendix. 3 to 4 liters of noxious, toxic stomach contents are spilled spreading bacteria throughout the belly and causing peritonitis. The pain steadily worsens with vomiting and a rising pulse. He may begin to improve deceptively before collapsing with a tender rigid abdomen. Breathing is shallow and he looks, and is, deathly.

Rx: morphine (D.1.4), cephalosporin (D.2.1), metronidazole (D.2.3). Drip-and-suck; evacuate urgently.

HERNIA

Gut or omentum may protrude through the muscular abdominal wall, usually in the groin, following the strain of carrying heavy loads. The resulting hernia may slide back on lying down, with the help of firm manual pressure. But gut may be nipped off and become strangulated, gangrenous and perforated. The tense, tender swelling in the groin cannot be pushed back; the victim vomits copiously, has griping pains, a distended belly and is shocked.

> In a tent north of Dhaulagiri in the Himalayas I once came across a Tibetan lama who looked just like this. After a dose of morphine and a mug of "rakshi" spirits I tried to squeeze the hernia back — to no avail. With two Sherpas holding him down, some local anesthetic, another monk chanting mantras, and a small suture kit I operated on him, untwisted the bowel and sewed him up. Ten minutes later a thunderous fart announced our luck and his life. Such surgery is neither recommended nor approved by the medical insurance agencies.

TESTICLE

Sudden pain without a story of injury is likely to be due either to acute inflammation or to torsion of the testicle, which must be untwisted urgently.

Act: support the scrotum in a tight pair of underpants well-padded with cotton-wool. Cautiously and gently attempt to unwind the torsion, and don't make him laugh.

Rx: cephalosporin (D.2.1).

PILES (HEMORRHOIDS)

Piles occur from straining at stool or carrying heavy loads, especially at high altitudes, with consequent overbreathing; the pressure within the abdomen rises causing piles to pop out. Always uncomfortable and inconvenient when prolapsed, they feel like grapes or varicose veins at the anal margin and can be very painful. Bright blood appears on the toilet paper after passing stool, and there is slimy, itchy discharge.

Act: have troublesome piles shrunk by a surgeon's needle (surprisingly painless) before setting out on a trip. If already embarked take bran to soften the stool, and drink enough fluid to prevent constipation. Avoid morphine or codeine. Keep scrupulously clean because soiling with feces causes maddening itch.

Rx: bismuth subgallate (D.9.5) hemorrhoidal cream or suppository.

Push prolapsed piles back inside the anus quickly to avoid them swelling and staying out. Dropping your trousers at 7,000m (20,000ft) in a blizzard is bad enough, but having prolapsed piles as well is the ultimate misery.

11 ABDOMINAL INJURY

The abdomen houses 9m (28ft) of gut and several major organs; liver, spleen, kidneys, bladder. The entire cavity and the organs themselves are enveloped in a thin membrane of peritoneum, which allows gut to move around without friction. Peritoneum senses pain when stretched or irritated by noxious fluids or blood.

Serious injury to the abdomen, whether blunt (closed) or sharp (penetrating), may cause internal bleeding or leakage of gut contents, feces, pus or urine; any or all of these cause peritonitis. So be alert, even after a minor blow, for possible internal mischief not immediately manifest. Surgery is the treatment for most abdominal injuries.

Closed abdominal injury

Ask: about the nature of the object causing the injury, and the way the accident happened, for example, falling across a rock, or onto an ice-axe.

SIGNS AND SYMPTOMS OF CLOSED ABDOMINAL INJURY
OR ABDOMINAL MISCHIEF
Pain: varies greatly; if severe the victim lies quite still. Pain is usually felt first around the umbilicus but spreads and settles in the region of the injured organ. Noxious fluids in contact with the under surface of the diaphragm irritate the phrenic nerve referring pain to one or both shoulder tips.

Tenderness: is general with guarding over the injured organs. If peritonitis spreads the abdominal muscles feel rigid, like pressing on a board. Further pressure causes pain, especially when the examining hand is suddenly removed (rebound tenderness).

Shock: is always present after internal bleeding. The victim is pale, sweaty and cold with a rapid, feeble pulse. If there is no external bleeding look to the abdomen for the cause. Shock is uncommon in head injury.

Vomiting: preceded by nausea is a constant sign of abdominal mischief, especially peritonitis. Bleeding from the stomach is rare in abdominal trauma so if bright-red fresh blood appears in the vomit look for an injured nose, mouth or tongue.

Blood in the urine: damage to the kidneys or bladder is likely; blood at the end of the penis suggests injury to the urethra.

Breathing is quiet, using the lower chest with the abdomen held still.

Act: Reassure; if the victim is flippant about an injury you suspect is not trivial, warn him of possible serious consequences and get help as soon as possible.

Rest: completely and allow only sips of water by mouth as he may vomit: but a dry person is a restless one. Don't worry about fluid in his stomach; this is the hospital anesthetist's problem, not yours, and he can deal with it.

Record: all observations every half-hour on paper, especially the pulse rate and any change in his condition.

Rx: morphine (D.1.4) relieves pain and allays anxiety, but it causes vomiting; so give promethazine (D.3.1) as well. Do not withold analgesics for fear of masking pain from the doctor who will try to diagnose him later; the effects of morphine can always be reversed with naloxone (D.1.5). Always write the drug name, the dose, and the time given, on a label and attach it to the victim for the information of the receiving doctor.

Infection: the stage is set because blood is an ideal medium for growing bugs, and spilt intestinal contents are teeming with bacteria. Give large doses of broad spectrum antibiotics (D.2).

SPECIFIC CLOSED INJURIES
Spleen: quite trivial force can rupture the spleen. When the lower left ribs are fractured the underlying spleen may be impaled. So always suspect abdominal organ rupture after a chest injury, especially on the left. Progressive severe bleeding with shock is

usual after rupture, but silent symptomless bleeding may continue from several hours to 3 weeks beneath the enfolding capsule which stretches and suddenly bursts, spilling blood into the peritoneum. The victim becomes deeply shocked. Therefore anyone suffering an abdominal injury in the wilderness, however mild, should be evacuated because of the danger of secondary hemorrhage.

Liver: caused by a crushing blow to the upper abdomen or fracture of the lower right ribs. Minor tears often stop bleeding; in massive injury it continues unabated. Occasionally a subcapsular hematoma develops (similar to the spleen) with sudden catastrophic bleeding after a delay of some hours.

Kidney: caused by a direct blow in the loin or flank, possibly with a fracture of the 12th rib. Pain is local when bleeding is contained within the capsule of the kidney, and blood is usually seen in the urine (hematuria). Many cases resolve with rest alone.

Urethra: a tear occurs when a fractured segment of pelvis to which the urethra is tethered, is pulled apart, or after falling astride a solid object like a tree or onto a rock. The victim, most commonly a man, has severe pain in the crotch, which is badly bruised between the scrotum and the anus. Look for fresh blood at the end of the penis. He will be unable to pass urine. The bladder becomes distended some hours later, can be felt above the pubic bone, and is very uncomfortable. Instead of passing down the damaged urethra, urine and blood may spread up into the muscle planes of the lower abdomen or of the perineum, which readily become infected.

Rx: broad spectrum antibiotic (D.2) immediately. No harm can come from 24 hours of inactivity, but a lot of damage may ensue from attempting to pass a catheter because the few remaining strands by which the urethra can re-canalize itself may be broken. Leave the catheter to a waterworks specialist because meddling now may make it irreparable later.

If far from help and if his bladder swells after waiting 24 hours, plunge a wide bore sterile needle through the cleansed skin of the abdominal wall in the mid-line 2cm (1″) above the pubic bone at least 5cm (2″) deep (bladder is close against abdominal wall with nothing else intervening at this point), and let urine spurt out. Repeated stabs, perhaps every 8 hours or whenever the bladder appears full, are less likely to cause infection than leaving an indwelling needle or canula.

Bladder: rupture is rare.

Act: supra-pubic drainage (as above) and Rx: antibiotics (D.2) will tide him over until he can reach a surgeon.

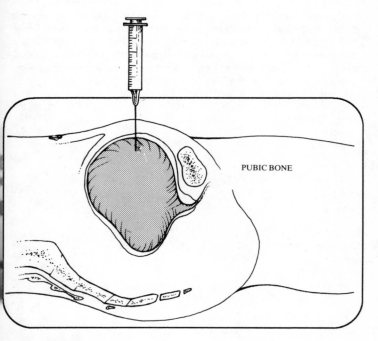

PUBIC BONE

Supra-pubic bladder drain

Open abdominal injury

In the rare event of an open wound from a knife, ice-axe or gun-shot, guts or fatty omentum may protrude — a horrendous sight. Do not try to push them back inside, but cover the wound with a clean, preferably sterile, damp dressing. If the instrument that caused the injury is still in the wound and if you can reach help quickly, leave it there as, like the Dutch boy's finger in the dike, it may be plugging the hole. However, if it is in a major blood vessel it may wriggle free during transport, and this would be fatal. So you may have to take a chance and remove it.

A small puncture wound of the skin should cause as much anxiety as an obvious gash. You can only guess whether the instrument has nicked the skin and penetrated muscle, or whether it has pierced an internal organ. A long sharp object, like a knife, which punctures the skin can be withdrawn leaving barely a mark, but punctured bowel may seal over temporarily and leak noxious fluid later — with fatal outcome. Most surgeons assume that a puncture wound has penetrated the abdominal cavity until proved otherwise, and operate forthwith.

12   WOUNDS AND POISONS

This chapter assumes a medical kit at least as comprehensive as
that listed on pages 21-27. Improvising with imagination will have
to supplement any missing items.

Superficial wounds

ABRASIONS
Grazes, scrapes, and minor burns must be cleaned with copious
water and soap; dilution is the solution to pollution. Superficial
wounds heal best when left open to fresh air, allowing them to dry
and form a scab — Nature's dressing. Avoid unctions that keep a
wound moist; if there are signs of infection an antibiotic by mouth
is preferable to antibiotic ointment.

If the wound has to be covered because of oozing, infection or if
the site is unsuitable for exposure, use a sterile gauze dressing
held in place with any kind of tape.

CUTS
A small sterile dressing (Band-Aid, Elastoplast) should suffice for
cover. If the wound edges are cleanly cut, close apposition will
give the least eventual, scar. Use sterile paper strips (Steri-strips)
or butterfly dressings. Paint tincture of benzoin on the
surrounding skin to make it tacky and adhesive. Carefully place
the strips, alternating the direction of pull of each, so as to bring
the edges of the wound together and keep the tension equal down
the length of the wound. For awkward places — between the
fingers, around the ankle — "Anchor Dressings" conform closely
to uneven contours.

BLISTERS
Blisters are usually caused by ill-fitting, or stiff boots. Cover a
sore "hot-spot" immediately to prevent it rubbing and becoming a
fluid-filled blister. Paint the skin around with tincture of benzoin
and apply tape directly onto the skin well above and below the

rubbed area. Use white surgical tape, silver aluminum duct tape or moleskin. To take the pressure off a large blister cut a doughnut from moleskin and place the hole right over the bleb. Leave the tape in place for a week if necessary. Do not burst small blisters; if large and likely to burst with the rubbing of a boot, clean the skin and puncture the edge in order to release the fluid, using a needle sterilized by holding it in a flame till red-hot. Leave the overlying skin in place as a dressing. Clean with soap and water, and dress.

Deep wounds

LACERATIONS
Cut, torn, or mangled tissue is best cleaned and left gaping to heal from the bottom of the wound outwards. Closing can be done later if necessary (delayed primary healing) as is done in war wounds. This is much safer than trying to suture wounds in the wilds where sterility is impossible, and because sutures themselves act as a foreign body in the wound and a focus for infection. For this reason no instructions are given in this book on how to suture, although a simple enough procedure in itself. Nature does a marvellous job with most wounds provided there is no infection; should She fail, a plastic surgeon can tidy up the scar much later.

PUNCTURE WOUNDS
Although tiny on the surface, puncture wounds may have a long track and there's no telling how deeply they penetrate. Beware — those of the chest and abdomen are potential minefields, so seek a surgeon quickly.

GUNSHOT WOUNDS
Leave the bullet or the pellets in place unless they are easily extracted.

Bleeding (hemorrhage)

Severe external bleeding will almost always stop with firm pressure directly on the wound, raising the injured part and resting the

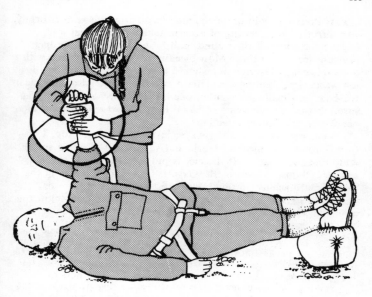

Press and elevate to stop bleeding

victim. Deep internal hemorrhage is a much more serious matter usually needing surgery.

An average adult male has about 5½ liters of circulating blood, a female, 4½ liters. Each can afford to lose about 1 liter before anemia and shock are noticed. Loss of more than ⅓ of the total blood volume can kill. Children tolerate blood loss less well than adults. The difference between bleeding from arteries and veins is academic; severe bleeding whatever its source must be stopped urgently.

Bleeding may halt spontaneously because muscle and elastic tissue in blood vessel walls contract, shed blood forms fibrin clot (but rarely within an undamaged vessel), or hidden bleeding in a closed space either closes off vessels in tissue planes between muscles by the build-up of fluid tension, or bleeding continues unabated into the cavity.

Act: Pressure — in order to stop bleeding press steadily, firmly and directly on a dressing of absorbent material placed well beyond the edges of the wound; and be prepared to keep up pressure for a long time. Most bleeding will eventually stop with pressure alone. The dressing should preferably be sterile but do not waste time hunting for a sterile dressing; any reasonably clean material, especially if recently ironed, will suffice and speed may save the victim from dying of blood loss. A doctor can worry later about any subsequent infection.

Do not remove soaked dressings; just pack more on top. Clot forms around the mesh of fabric and seals small bleeding vessels and oozing capillaries. If the clot is pulled off bleeding will start again. Cellulose gelatin mesh (Oxycel, Gelfoam) dissolves in the wound and hastens clotting. Wrap absorbent stretchy tensor bandage to keep the wound packing in place. This will splint the area and avoid movement that might restart bleeding.

Pressure points are only useful for students of anatomy. Valuable time may be lost while searching for them. Do not take a wide, blind suture needle bite to close off the wound because the suture will be a focus for infection, and nerves and other structures in the depths of the wound may be damaged.

Tourniquets may obstruct veins without controlling arterial bleeding. They may be tied and then forgotten causing obstruction to blood supply and gangrene of the limb beyond. Pressure may damage nerves. Pain from a tourniquet causes restlessness. In the rare event of a tourniquet being necessary because other methods have failed to control bleeding, for example, traumatic amputation of the hand, release the tourniquet every 45 minutes, mark a large T on the victim's forehead with a pen or lip-stick, and record on a label tied round his neck the time when it was applied. On the rare occasion when a large artery is severed and bleeding cannot be controlled by pressure or a tourniquet, it may be necessary to clamp the ends with a hemostat and tie off the vessel with a suture.

Cleaning — wash the wound with copious soap and water to get rid of grease and grime. Plentiful washing gives bacteria less chance to survive and cause infection. Pick out dirt with forceps but do not scrub because tissue will be further damaged. Antiseptic solutions can cause chemical irritation and are no better than soap and water. The rescuer's hands should be washed as meticulously as the wound.

Dressings — place a sterile dressing next to the wound. Compressed wound dressings are ideal; tightly packaged womens' sanitary napkins are cheap and available. Ironed cloth, unopened toilet paper or paper tissues are all but sterile. To increase the bulk of a dressing any clean absorbent cloth, like a shirt, can be slapped on top.

Paraffin gauze squares (Jelonet) are useful for covering oozing wounds; the gauze may be impregnated with antibiotic (Sofratulle). Stretchy, clear plastic kitchen wrap can be applied straight onto a wound or a burn if a closed dressing is required. A mangled limb can be wrapped temporarily in a plastic bag taped closed to the skin at both ends.

TETANUS PREVENTION
Anyone planning a trip should be up-to-date with tetanus immunization; protection lasts 5 years. After a wound an anti-tetanus booster dose of 0.5-1.0ml should be sought from a doctor, who should always ask about previous reactions to anti-tetanus serum, and if in doubt should not give it.

Infection

An inflamed wound looks red, swells, feels hot and throbs painfully. The body is thereby mobilizing its defenses of white blood cells, which flow along dilated blood vessels into the area in order to combat bacteria. An infected wound has pus in it made of gobbled-up bugs and dead tissue which coalesce into a boil or abscess.

LOCALIZED INFECTION (BOIL OR ABSCESS)
A tense infected swelling usually comes to a head and forms a white or yellow boil with a soft center of pus, which may discharge on its own. A red streak caused by inflamed lymph channels, often leads towards the heart; swelling occurs in regional lymph nodes that drain the infected area — in the groin from the leg, in the armpit from the arm.

Act: heat encourages pus to gather. Every 6 hours soak the area in warm salt water or apply a hot compress of cloth dipped in boiling water and wrung out. Honey, baking soda or glycerine magnesium sulphate paste draws out pus hygroscopically.

Where there's pus let it out. When an abscess has a soft centre indicating liquid pus, lance it to allow the pus to drain. But beware of draining an abscess before it is "ripe" because it will be painful and produce no pus. A quick stab into the stretched skin over a ripe abscess causes little pain especially if ice or snow are applied for 5 minutes beforehand. Make the incision deep and long so the hole will not seal over and nullify the good work of drainage. Sudden release of pus under pressure relieves pain instantly. If the hole is deep pack it with a wick of sterile gauze.

Rx: cephalosporin (D.2.1) as soon as a wound becomes red and inflamed. Avoid antibiotic ointments which may cause sensitivity reactions.

SPREADING INFECTION (CELLULITIS)

The skin around a wound looks red and angry, and feels hot and hard owing to swelling. Regional lymph nodes swell.

Act: immobilize the part and elevate it to reduce swelling.

Rx: antibiotics (D.2) i/v if possible, in double dose.

GENERALIZED INFECTION (BLOOD POISONING OR SEPTICEMIA)

High fever and chills in the presence of infection suggest septicemia — a serious complication which needs urgent medical help.

Rx: antibiotics (D.2) i/v if possible, in double dose, and rest.

WOOD SLIVER

Pull the sliver out with forceps or tweezers, but it may be very difficult to find even if judged to be just under the skin. Inject 1ml of local anesthetic lignocaine (D.17.1) directly into the area. If the sliver won't come out soak in hot water and try again but don't damage tissue by persevering. If left alone pus will eventually form around a sliver, which will extrude with pressure of a developing abscess.

METAL FOREIGN BODY

Leave well alone unless easily removed with tweezers. A broken-off needle fragment may remain inert and harmless for years. Removing it surgically, even with x-ray help, is notoriously difficult.

FISH HOOK REMOVAL

Push the hook onwards until it pierces the skin again. Cut off the barbed end with pliers, cupping a hand over the cutters to prevent the barb flying into your own eye. Then withdraw the shank of the hook by the way it went in. If pliers are unavailable hold the eye of the hook down against the skin, loop fishline or string around the hook, and jerk sharply along the plane of the skin surface thereby tearing it out.

BRUISES

Bruises occur when blood is shed under the skin. When the blood breaks down with time the overlying skin turns the colors of the rainbow.

SUPERFICIAL BRUISES

Black eye: blood collects in the loose tissues around the eye but enclosed by the margin of the bony orbit. It will subside with ice and time.

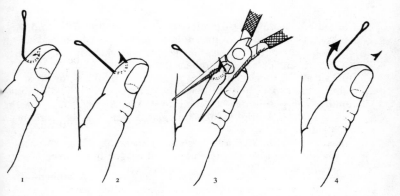

Removing fish-hook

Finger-nail blood blister (subungual hematoma): when a finger-nail is bashed or a boulder drops on a toe, a tense, painful bruise forms at the root of the nail; it turns black, is soggy on pressure, and is excruciatingly painful.

Act: heat an opened metal paper-clip held in forceps or pliers over a stove or a propane lighter flame (candle flame is not hot enough). When the paper-clip end is red-hot, push it cautiously into the middle of the moon of the nail over the bruise so it burns right through the nail but not into the nail bed. The resulting sizzling smells like a smithy. Old, dark blood spurts out and the sun shines again from the face of the victim, who will be your instant friend, unless you have plunged too deep. Alternatively, drill the base of the nail by rotating a penknife blade.

Deep bruise (hematoma): a painful swelling can arise from blood pooling in muscle over a point of injury. Rest, elevation and ice may be all that is necessary for it to subside. If the bruise is tense and seems filled with fluid, clean the skin carefully and push the largest available needle into the swelling in order to drain the pooled serum.

Poisons

INHALED GAS

Carbon monoxide is a by-product of most camping stoves and the gas can accumulate in an unventilated tent, especially if sealed with snow cover. In cold weather people may camp in their vans, leaving the engine running to heat the cab into which exhaust fumes leak. Carbon monoxide is odorless; a small amount in a tightly-closed space gives little warning of its presence and can kill rapidly. The victim may be found unconscious, very pale and with luck still alive. A bright-pink skin color is seen in severe carbon monoxide poisoning.

Act: remove the victim to fresh air immediately, keep an open airway and give assisted breathing, with oxygen if possible. A vicious headache will develop during recovery.

SWALLOWED POISONS

Most drugs swallowed accidentally or intentionally must be got rid

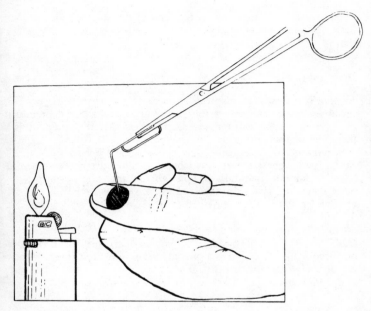

Draining fingernail

of before they are absorbed by the blood stream. Give an emetic
made with milk followed by a strong salty drink, and stick a
finger down the throat. A stomach wash-out is the most effective
way of evacuating poison provided it is done within 4 hours of
swallowing; but it can be dangerous if not done skillfully,
preferably with mechanical suction at hand. Corrosives, acids and
industrial poisons are best left lying where they are because they
will burn the esophagus if vomited. Dilute them with large
volumes of water and/or milk or white of egg.

   Act: stomach wash-out only if the person is conscious and can
protect his own airway. Lie him on one side and pass a well-
lubricated tube, at least 1cm diameter, down the throat into the
stomach. Attach a funnel, hold it high and pour in a liter of

water. Lower the funnel below the level of the stomach and let the fluid run out. Repeat until the washings are clear — at least 6 times.

Drug abuse

Alcohol is the most common drug used, and abused; it loosens social restraints and gives a false sense of bravado, but depresses the nervous system and impairs all reactions. Alcohol compounds the effect of some other drugs.

Strange behavior, especially after a prolonged boring spell in camp, may suggest a person is stoned on other drugs. Prevent him harming himself, maintain an open airway, talk him down in a quiet place and give calm reassurance. Do not leave him unattended until he has emerged from his trip.

COMMONLY ABUSED DRUGS:

Hallucinogens — LSD (acid), PCP (angel dust), psilocybin (magic mushrooms) cause hallucinations, agitation and excitement. Pupils are dilated, except with PCP.

Rx: lorazepam (D.5.1).

Narcotics — heroin, morphine, codeine, meperidine, methadone cause seizures, coma and depressed breathing. Pupils are pinpoint.

Rx: naloxone (D.1.5) reverses narcotics and restores breathing. Vomiting may need suction. Seizures are controlled with lorazepam (D.5.1) preferably given i/v. The victim must be watched closely for 24 hours because his breathing may quit, needing resuscitation and more naloxone.

Cannabis group — marijuana, hashish: eyes are bloodshot, pupils unchanged and the pulse races.

Nervous system depressants "downers" — barbiturates, diazepam (Valium), chlordiazepoxide (Librium), glutethamide (Doriden), methalqualone (Quaaludes): the depressant effect is increased by alcohol. Severe withdrawal symptoms occur.

Nervous system stimulants "uppers" — amphetamines (speed), cocaine, anti-obesity drugs: pupils are dilated but react to light, breathing is shallow, and pulse races. Seizures can occur.

Rx: lorazepam (D.5.1)

Anti-cholinergics — atropine (belladonna), tricyclic anti-depressants, Jimson weed, henbane, mandrake: pupils are dilated and fixed, pulse races, skin is dry.

Other poisons

FUNGI

Avoid all wild mushrooms unless you understand them. Violent vomiting, diarrhea and abdominal cramps come on 8 hours after eating the fungi.

Act: give repeated cups of hot tea, an emetic of salty water, Epsom salts and empty the bowel by a soap and water enema.

BOTULISM

Home-canned or bottled food may harbor Clostridium botulinum. Seal meat is notorious. Double vision, various muscle paralyses and abdominal discomfort come on after 6 to 24 hours often in several participants of the same meal.

Act: seek expert help urgently. Rx: [botulinus antitoxin] 50,000U i/m stat.

13   BURNS AND HEAT INJURY

Sunburn is a common painful nuisance. The sun is a stealthy enemy; it reflects strongly off water, sand and snow. Ultra-violet rays penetrate hazy cloud, and the higher the altitude the more they burn; each 300m altitude rise adds 4% to the rays' intensity. Those with fair skin, red hair or freckles are more liable to sunburn. Tanning is the best skin protection but people tan at varying speed. Rationing sunlight on the skin is the cheapest, most effective way to avoid sunburn and to tan. Wear a wide-brimmed hat or a peaked cap with a neck cover. Sun-glasses should have blinker side-pieces and nose-shields. Lips and noses burn, especially on the underside, from ultra-violet light reflected off snow. Unlike sunbathing on the beach it is more difficult to cut down the length of sun exposure in the wilderness. Falling asleep in the sun is a sure way to fry, and even a sola topi worn at midday won't save mad dogs or Englishmen.

Sun creams and lotions act as a screen to the burning parts of the ultra-violet spectrum; none speed "le bronzage", and with excessive sun they just act as fat for frying. Para-aminobenzoic acid is the base of most sunscreens. The Sun Protection Factor (SPF) should be marked on the bottle from 1 to 20; the higher the number, the more the protection.

Act: find shade if skin goes shrimp-pink, and feels prickly and hot. Baking soda compresses or calamine soothe.

Rx: anti-histamines (D.3) allay itching; avoid topical local anesthetic and anti-histamine creams which can cause sensitivity reactions. Badly burnt skin goes bright lobster-red and blisters.

betamethasone steroid cream (D.11.1)

paracetamol (D.1.1) for fever. Severe general body upset (hyperthermia see p. 190) with headache, vomiting and fainting may ensue. Cool with ice and fanning

FLAME BURN

Open air: flame burns and scalds go hand-in-hand with hot cooking pans, boiling water, and hot fat. The flash of flame from ignited gasoline or propane passes in a second; the skin turns brown or black, but the burn will probably be superficial and heal within a couple of weeks. Flaming clothing continues to burn the skin for several seconds, often causing a deep burn which takes weeks, or months, to heal and may need skin-grafting. Some synthetic fabrics like nylon and polypropylene melt and burn deeply. Fireproof synthetic materials are labelled as such. Wool and natural fiber do not hold flame, so the burn is delayed in reaching the skin; but wool keeps boiling water in contact with the skin, thus prolonging the scalding time. Boiling water and frying pan fat aflame on bare skin often burn deeply.

Enclosed space: explosions within an enclosed space like a tent, snow cave, or camper van produce hot gases which are inhaled, burning the air passages and lungs — often fatally. Liquid propane gas is heavier than air and, when spilled, settles on the floor. If ignited by a match, a spark, or another stove it explodes.

FRICTION BURNS

Deep friction burns to the hands, neck and back can occur when a climber tries to hold a falling companion, or when roping down.

ELECTRICAL BURNS

Deeper and more extensive than at first sight, electrical burns heal slowly, especially at the point where the current enters and leaves the body.

Lightning: is a danger on mountain summits and ridges, and when sitting under a tree or other conductor. It usually strikes the head causing unconsciousness, and deafness for 1 to 2 weeks after. If the heart is struck the victim may die of ventricular fibrillation. With a direct strike the burn spreads over the skin surface making a fern-like pattern; an indirect burn is caused by superheated air near the object struck.

Car battery: burns may occur when booster cables are connected wrongly.

Chemical burns: are usually caused by lime or acid. Car batteries may explode violently if a spark ignites escaping hydrogen gas. Severity of a burn is assessed by measuring the burned body surface area (b.s.a.) irrespective of depth, according to the "rule of 9s". The palm area of the victim's hand, not the rescuer's, is 1% b.s.a.

Minor burns (less than 15% b.s.a.) heal unaided.

Major burns (more than 15% b.s.a. in adults) are a threat to life with consequences stretching far beyond the burn wound itself. In children a major burn is more than 10% b.s.a. because children have a greater body surface in relation to their weight.

MINOR BURNS should be immediately washed with copious water and are generally best left open to the air to dry or covered with a small sterile dressing, if such is appropriate. They usually heal quickly and completely so long as there is no infection.

MAJOR BURNS cause two main problems, tissue damage and fluid loss; together these lead to "burn shock" similar to the shock that follows severe bleeding. Emotional shock — fear, pain, and fainting — that follows the burning accident compound and worsen clinical shock. Major burns always need fluid replacement.

Tissue damage

A burn is a wound; the depth of tissue destroyed is important in determining the time a wound will take to heal, and whether skin-grafting will be necessary.

DEPTH OF BURN

Partial-thickness (superficial): burn penetrates to, and harms to a variable extent, the germinal epithelium where are generated new cells that spread out to form new epidermal skin. Partial-thickness burns usually heal unaided in 7-21 days if kept clean and dry. Infection delays healing and may convert a partial-thickness burn into one of full-thickness.

Full-thickness (deep): extend through the germinal layer of cells destroying nerves and blood vessels, hair follicles and sweat glands that lie in that layer. The skin will not regenerate on its own and

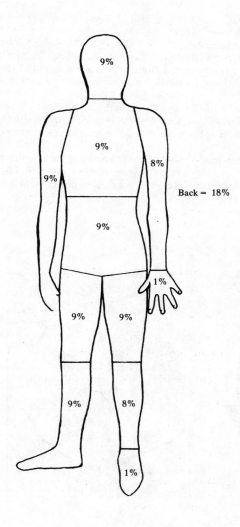

Rule of 9s

will usually need skin-grafting. The color of burned skin is a poor guide to burn depth.

Better tests are:

Pinprick: if the victim can feel the prick of a sterile needle firm enough to draw blood (light touch is not enough) the burn is superficial. In a full-thickness burn nerves are destroyed so pain is absent.

Pressure: if the skin feels leathery and firm on pressure it is deeply burned — a useful test in scalds where the skin looks pink. If the color returns quickly when pressure is removed, the burn is superficial.

Exuded plasma and coagulated tissue form a slough, which hardens to a dry crust (eschar) if left open to the air and kept clean of infection. Healing goes on under the crust which

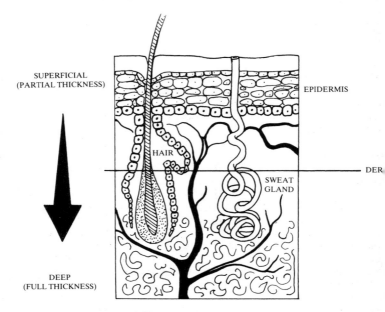

Burn skin depth

eventually separates leaving a raw area (granulation tissue). Early skin grafting in hospital can prevent the hideous disabling deformities that are a common sequel to major burns.

Act: cool; immediately douse any burn, whatever the cause, with cold water or snow for at least 10 minutes. Cooling halts burning and eases pain. Before focusing attention on the victim's burn wound attend to the airway and treat pain.

Airway: to lose a burn victim from airway block is tragic because it is usually avoidable (see p. 47).

An endotracheal tube should be passed early rather than late. A tracheotomy may be needed on reaching hospital — never in the field.

Pain: not only is pain unpleasant but also it aggravates shock. Reassure the victim and give enough drugs to kill the pain. A superficial burn will usually hurt because the nerve-endings in the epidermis are intact; they are destroyed in a deep burn which may be free of pain.

Rx: morphine (D.1.4).

Managing a major burn in the wilds will be very difficult. The ideal treatment is explained here, knowing you will not be able to carry it out fully. Do not despair just because you are in remote wilderness several days, or weeks, away from help. Ingenuity and common sense must prevail.

THE BURN WOUND
Whatever the cause, the immediate care of the burn wound is the same; refinements in treatment come later.

Cool: douse the burned area in cold water or snow.

Undress: remove clothing in order to examine the full extent of the burn. If charred fabric sticks to the skin leave it in place because pulling it away may restart bleeding; it will be sterile anyway because of the heat. Remove rings and jewelry which may constrict the circulation after swelling.

Wash: with copious soap and water. With sterile forceps remove

dead tissue that comes away easily. Irrigate chemical burns
(especially lime in the eyes) with plain water for at least 10
minutes.

Record: draw a careful diagram of the area of the burn (rule of
9s), and the depth of burning (pinprick test) in order to follow the
progress of healing during the long days ahead. Ask how the
accident occurred and what steps were taken to extinguish the
cause of the burn.

When exposed to open air, provided it remains absolutely clean,
a burn wound will dry forming a crusting scab (eschar or
carapace) under which healing proceeds free from bacteria. But
since open exposure will be impossible out in the wilderness the
wound needs to be dressed.

Dressing: cover the wound with clean, sterile, dry linen or non-
stick dressing. A dressing acts as a mechanical barrier to infection
and absorbs exudate from the wound, allowing it to dry and start
healing. Apply a pad of absorbent cotton-batten on top of the
dressing in order to soak up exuded fluid. Two layers of plain
paraffin gauze may be used next to the burn. The dressing should
extend at least a handbreadth beyond the edge of the burn.
Finally, wrap a crepe bandage evenly over the dressing, firmly
enough to keep it in place but not so tight as to restrict
circulation. Do not smear the burn with butter, burn creams, or
patent potions which confuse the picture and make dressings stick
fast. Avoid antibiotic creams because they encourage the growth of
resistant bacteria.

If there is no immediate chance of reaching help a burn
dressing can be left in place for up to a week provided it remains
dry and free of infection. Repeated peeking at the wound lays
open a path for infection to enter. As soon as plasma soaks
through the dressing replace the outer absorbent packing only,
leaving the immediate dressing in place. If it smells foul, has a
pussy discharge, if pain and redness develop in skin away from
the burn, or if the victim's temperature rises, undo the dressing
completely and start again because these are signs of infection.

Blisters: leave a small blister alone and use a moleskin doughnut to keep off pressure while it heals. Leave large blisters intact if possible because they form a skin roof and a good sterile enclosure. If the blister is in a place that will rub it will break anyway, so puncture the blebs with a sterile needle or blade. Careful lancing on the first day can be quite painless. Keep the resulting open wound scrupulously clean as infection can easily creep in. If blisters break by themselves and become infected they are very painful.

  Rx: antibiotic (D.2) for at least 10 days if infection supervenes.
  codeine (D.1.3) or morphine (D.1.4). dressing changes are agony, so give a strong pain-killer before starting.
  tetanus toxoid; get a booster dose as soon as help is reached.

All treatment is aimed towards keeping the burn wound clean and avoiding infection. Skin-grafting may be needed to treat areas of full-thickness burning in hospital. If the wound is clean this can be done soon after arrival.

Fluid loss

Damaged capillaries leak plasma, the fluid portion of blood, which exudes from the raw burn surface, forms blisters under the outer layers of the skin, and collects in swollen tissues. The body compensates for loss of plasma from a burn by withdrawing fluid from regions where it is not needed instantly. Vessels in the periphery of the skin and in the gut clamp down so blood pools in the central circulation, and compulsive thirst and drinking makes up for some of the lost fluid — all the early signs of shock. .

After a major burn plasma must be replaced quickly, if possible intravenously, in order to avoid shock; the longer the delay the worse the outcome. Severe bleeding causes immediate shock in proportion to the blood lost; but burn shock develops slowly over several hours owing to accumulated toxic products of tissue destruction and plasma loss. The victim appears deceptively well soon after the accident and then deteriorates over the next 24 to 36 hours. Some red cells are destroyed in the scorched skin, others pass into the circulation and fragment later leading to anemia. The breakdown products of blood cells lodge in the kidney and give the urine a red-brown color.

Act: measure the burned area accurately according to the rule of 9s paying attention only to the area, not the depth of burning. Replace fluid according to your estimate of the victim's needs based on his condition.

After a major burn an intravenous drip is the best way of restoring fluid balance. If you are out in the boondocks other routes must be considered; unlike intravenous fluid they cannot overload the circulation but are less efficient.

ORAL

The victim should drink 3 liters daily if possible, giving small sips rather than big gulps in order to avoid vomiting. Water will do, but the WHO formula (D.18) will replace enough electrolyte, glucose, and water to keep the victim of a 50% burn alive.

RECTAL

A greased wide-bore tube is inserted as high up the rectum as possible, preferably about 15cm (7″) from the anus. Fluid of any sort is run in as fast as the victim can retain it without overflow.

NASO-GASTRIC

If the victim cannot drink, a greased 14mm diameter naso-gastric tube is passed into the stomach via the nose (difficult sometimes to turn the bend at the back of the pharynx), or through the mouth (may make him gag and vomit). To tell when the tube is lying in the stomach, watch for fluid in an attached funnel start to flow; gurgling can be heard with a stethoscope or an ear placed over the upper abdomen.

SUBCUTANEOUS

The needle of an intravenous apparatus is inserted under the loose skin on the front of the chest just below the clavicle or abdomen. The needle lies in the plane between skin and muscle where fluid spreads and is slowly absorbed; 3 liters should be put in each 24 hours.

INTRAVENOUS FLUID

Choose a large vein as the drip may have to last several days. The best replacement fluid is human plasma reconstituted with sterile water as it contains all the essential proteins; Ringer's lactate or normal saline will do temporarily.

The amount of fluid needed is 4 to 5 ml/kg body weight/24 hours at a rate of ½ the volume in the first 8 hour period, ¼ in each of the next 8 hour periods. This relates to the time of the burn and therefore initial fluid replacement must catch up and may have to be given rapidly. Thereafter give enough fluid to produce 30-50ml of urine each hour.

Special burn sites

FACE, EYELIDS, EYES
Most face burns can be left exposed to the air. But the lax tissues
of the lids swell and may close the victim's eyes; he needs
reassurance that he is not going blind. Burns of the cornea, the
window of the eye, are uncommon because blinking usually occurs
before the flame reaches the eye. Corrosive chemicals must be
washed out thoroughly with water until every particle has gone.
Lids may retract as the burn dries, so the cornea becomes exposed
and an ulcer will follow. Snow-blindness is an ultra-violet burn of
the cornea.

Rx: chloramphenicol ointment (D.12.1) into the eye twice daily
to lubricate the lids and stave off infection and 2% homatropine
drops (D.12.3) twice daily to keep the pupil dilated and ease
painful spasm of the iris. Use dark glasses rather than a pad and
bandage which can be very uncomfortable.

If the lips, tongue or the nostril hairs are scorched after an
explosion the victim has probably inhaled burning gas; and the
outcome is poor. The larynx and trachea will swell making the
voice husky at first, followed by croaking when the airway is
blocked. A lung burn usually leads to pneumonia and ultimately
to breathing failure and death.

CHEST AND NECK
If the burn is circumferential a crust, like a breast-plate of armor,
may form and restrict breathing.

> Make longitudinal cuts through the full thickness of burned skin to
> relieve breathing (see below — escharotomy).

HANDS
Burnt hands form nasty contracture deformities unless the hands
are kept moving while healing. Cover the whole hand liberally
with antibiotic cream and put it in a plastic bag taped at the
wrist. Encourage the victim to exercise his fingers continually to
prevent the skin hardening and the fingers becoming stiff. Elevate
the hand to reduce swelling. With a bagged hand the victim can
do a lot for himself without pain; a mitten over the top protects
the bag and looks less distasteful.

Deep burns of the circumference of limbs or fingers harden and the scab may contract like a ring and cut off the blood supply or restrict movement. Check by pin-prick for pain sensation; if absent, escharotomy is needed.

ESCHAROTOMY
This simple surgical procedure, though seemingly drastic, may be limb-saving. It could preserve the fingers after deep burns round the wrist, which heal with a tight constricting band. Make a deep knife cut through charred skin along the lateral sides of the limb or digits. The wound will spread apart owing to the pressure within. To be effective the cut must extend beyond the top and bottom of the eschar down into the unburned zone, which feels pain and may bleed. If the cuts are adequate, the swollen veins and mottled blue color of the skin return to a healthy pink. Where fingers are burned deeply to the tips all round, it is doubtful if escharotomy makes much difference.

Finally, do not delay evacuating the burned victim to hospital, as he will travel best immediately after the accident, before shock sets in. Do the best you can in the time while waiting for rescue. Reassure the victim that everything is being done to reach help urgently. Do not brush off his questions, but give a full reply. Let's hope optimism is warranted.

Heat injury

The body gains heat from its own basal metabolism, by exercise and from the environment; heat is lost by evaporation from sweating, conduction and convection.

HEAT EXHAUSTION
Heat exhaustion occurs when metabolic heat production increases greatly with exertion but thirst does not stimulate adequate drinking for replacement of fluid. It includes all forms of heat-induced water and salt depletion, short of heat stroke. Heat exhaustion can occur at modest temperatures, 16°C (60°F), if exercise is sufficiently vigorous. The risk is increased on a hot day, in bright sun, high humidity, calm wind and by wearing too much heavy, dark, impermeable clothing. Training to tolerate heat takes at least 10 days.

Look: the victim's temperature, measured rectally, is moderately raised, 39.5°C (103°F) to 42°C (107°F). He is very thirsty, sweats profusely, and has a headache and goose-flesh. He is faint, chilled, nauseated and unsteady. He may become mentally strange, convulse and fall unconscious, progressing to heat-stroke.

When exercising in the heat drink water more frequently than thirst dictates, enough to keep the urine clear (4 to 6 litres daily). When running, drink 250ml before, and every 15 to 30 minutes throughout the run. An adequate volume of water needs replacing immediately; salt and glucose can be added later. Avoid fancy electrolyte and sugar solutions during activity because they slow absorption of water from the bowel. However, if salt is not replaced later heat cramps may follow.

Act: cool the victim immediately. Rub ice or snow vigorously on his neck, abdomen, axillae and groins; sprinkle him with cold water to increase evaporation. Immerse his trunk in a stream, but cool his limbs as litle as possible because peripheral vessels will constrict, reducing heat loss.

Rx: 1 liter of 5% dextrose-saline intravenously over 30 minutes, or as much as he can tolerate by mouth.

HEAT-STROKE

Heat-stroke is a medical emergency and people die from it. Brain function is deranged owing to raised temperature. It can occur at relatively low air temperature if the exercise is vigorous enough and if the air is humid. The risk is increased in someone with a high fever and dehydration.

Look: the victim's rectal temperature is around 41°C (106°F); it may be a degree or two either side of this but heat-stroke cannot be diagnosed by temperature alone. Without warning he may become confused, delirious or comatose. The skin is still sweaty when he collapses but may become hot and dry 1 to 2 hours afterwards because of heat damage to the sweat glands.

Act: cool him immediately and thoroughly — it may be life-saving. Only stop cooling when the rectal temperature is 39°C (102°F) because it will drop the rest of the way on its own. With cooling he may start shivering, which may be very painful and need analgesics.

14 SUNDRY MEDICAL PROBLEMS

Coma
In an unconscious person who has neither story nor sign of head injury, consider other causes of unconsciousness. Look for a Medic-Alert bracelet or medallion. But remember that the victim may also have struck his head while falling unconscious.

EPILEPSY
The victim of an epileptic seizure may let out a sudden cry and fall to the ground. He twitches, jerks violently, rolls his eyes, froths at the mouth, bites his tongue and pees his pants. The seizure usually passes off in a few minutes. He wakes up, but then shortly after falls into a deep sleep of recovery, which can be mistaken for coma.

Act: prevent him from injuring himself. Do not wedge anything between his teeth in order to stop tongue-biting; if the teeth are clenched the victim is conscious enough to be able to safeguard his own airway.

Rx: lorazepam (D.5.1) 1 - 2mg; i/v would be most effective as an anti-convulsant, by mouth it acts very slowly. If he is a known epileptic on treatment, usually with [phenytoin], double the dose for a day and make sure he never forgets to take his pills. Have him checked by a doctor soon.

DIABETES
Diabetics do not produce enough insulin, the hormone that allows the body to burn glucose as fuel for energy. A severe diabetic requires a calculated amount of carbohydrate each day and insulin injections, usually given by himself. Insulin should always be carried by a diabetic because returning to camp may be delayed by a storm or travel problems. If more fuel is expected to be burned, as in a hard day's exercise, temporarily increase carbohydrate intake. Forgetting to do so may lead to either hypoglycemia (too little sugar) because there is insufficient carbohydrate for the insulin to work on; or diabetic pre-coma (too

much sugar) when insulin or oral diabetic medication needs to be increased. Either of these two conditions may cause a slide into coma. Distinguishing which is which is vital because their treatment is contrary.

	HYPOGLYCEMIA	DIABETIC PRE-COMA
onset	sudden in healthy	gradual in ill person
appearance	shocked, cool	normal
tongue & skin	moist	dry
breath smell	normal	ketones (acid drops)
urine taste	bitter	sweet
Rx:	glucose	insulin

DRUG OVERDOSE
Alcohol; the smell of the breath gives the story away (except vodka which is odorless). Narcotics, barbiturates, benzodiazepines, and other drug overdoses;
   Act: stomach wash-out (see p.139)

STROKE
Although usually restricted to older people the young may suffer strokes, especially as a complication of high altitude. The victim complains first of headache, then loses consciousness. The head and eyes turn to one side and he becomes paralysed on the opposite side of the body, partially or completely. Breathing is heavy with snoring and may be periodic (Cheyne-Stokes).
   Act: evacuate urgently for all the above serious conditions.

HEART ATTACK (myocardial infarction)
Severe chest pain, shock and rapid breathing occur. Coma is unusual. Heart attack needs pain relief.
   Rx: morphine (D.1.4). Rest and oxygen help cyanosis. If the heart stops, start rescue breathing and chest compression. Seek urgent medical help.

HEART and CHEST

The symptoms and signs of heart and chest illness frequently overlap. The person may complain of chest pain, irregular heartbeat, cough, or difficulty and shortness of breathing. Weigh the history and examination findings in order to reach a diagnosis. Only conditions reasonably likely to be encountered in the outdoors are described here.

HISTORY AND SYMPTOMS
Ask the person for any past history of heart or chest disease. Is he now taking any medications? Look for Medic-Alert bracelet or medallion. Allergies? Smoker? Overweight?

Chest pain — ask the nature of the pain and its manner of onset (sudden or gradual).

Sharp — described as stabbing or knife-like. Pain that is worsened on inspiration, usually on one side only, and often referred to the shoulder or abdomen probably arises from the lung surface (pleurisy). Pain precisely localized to one tender rib may be due to fracture. Chest wall pain is accentuated by movement.

Dull — also described as gripping, vise-like, crushing, constricting. Angina typically is pain, pressure or tightness in the center or left side of the chest, or deep behind the sternum, possibly referred to the shoulder or arms or up into the neck or jaw. It comes on with exertion and is relieved by rest, usually in someone with known heart disease. Heart attack (myocardial infarction) may be associated with shortness of breath and sweaty, nauseating shock.

Pulse — rapid and regular; may be due to paroxysmal atrial tachycardia (PAT) which can occur in healthy people and may cause an uncomfortable feeling behind the sternum like butterflies. It engenders anxiety but usually needs no treatment; rarely it may be serious and cause shock. Tachycardia may be caused by fever or oxygen lack (hypoxia) especially at altitude.
— rapid and irregular; suggests heart disease; if combined with chest pain think of myocardial infarction.

— Slow (bradycardia); many athletes run a pulse of less than 50 beats/minute. It can also occur in heart block from myocardial infarction.

Cough — sudden, violent coughing and choking may be due to an inhaled foreign body. A dry cough occurs in early bronchitis; later yellow or green sputum appears. Bright-red or rusty blood-flecked sputum suggests pneumonia, which is often accompanied by fever and rigors. Pulmonary edema causes a dry cough with no sputum, less commonly a moist cough with pink, frothy sputum. The dry air at altitude causes cough that is very irritating and may be so violent as to break a rib.

Shortness of breath (dyspnea) — upper airway obstruction may be accompanied by noisy, croupy, whooping stridor during inspiration. — air in the pleural cavity arises from collapse of lung (pneumothorax — spontaneous or traumatic), fluid comes from an effusion possibly after pneumonia.
— stiffness of the lung because of congestion or consolidation (pneumonia) or edema due to heart failure caused by myocardial infarction, is often accompanied by dyspnea on lying down and swelling of the ankles.

Wheeze — noisy wheezing and dyspnea especially during expiration, and sometimes with cyanosis, suggests asthma or bronchitis. An asthma attack may be provoked in someone who is susceptible by contact with an allergen, for example; pollen, dust, feathers, animal fur or certain foods. Other causes are chest infection (bronchitis or pneumonia) or emotional upset.

Sputum — if the spit is thick yellow or green, chest infection is present so:
   Rx: antibiotic (D.2)

EXAM

Heart

Look: for swelling of the ankles that pits on finger pressure and shows the imprint of sock elastic, indicating heart failure. Look for the color and nutrition of the skin of the extremities.

Raised jugular venous pressure indicates right heart failure.

Cyanosis — a bluish color of the skin and lips shows in full daylight, but can be missed in poor lighting of a colored tent. Weather-beaten, sun-tanned skin disguises cyanosis, so compare a healthy person with the sick one. Cyanosis occurs in two forms.

Peripheral: seen best in the beds of the finger-nails and the lips, is due to sluggish flow of cold blood. The color returns to normal pink on warming. The tongue remains pink. Peripheral cyanosis occurs in shock when the blood pressure falls due to circulatory failure.

Central: the tongue, lips and mucous membranes inside the mouth are blue and do not turn pink on re-warming.

Central cyanosis indicates serious disturbance of heart and lung function because of either inadequate ventilation, uneven distrubution of blood, decreased diffusion of oxygen or abnormal shunting of blood within the chambers of the heart. It is common at high altitude because of diminished oxygen (hypoxia) and excessive red blood cell production (polycythemia) and disappears on breathing 100% oxygen for 10 minutes.

Feel: the pulse and guage the blood pressure (or measure it with a sphygmomanometer). Light finger-touch can tell whether the pulse is full and bounding, or weak and thready.

The apex beat, if displaced to the left, shows an enlarged heart. The peripheral pulses: femoral, posterior tibial and dorsalis pedis, assess the peripheral circulation. Only a trained ear can interpret abnormal heart sounds and rhythms.
  Listen to the heart sounds, preferably with a stethoscope, if not, with an ear placed against the victim's chest.

Chest

Look: at the chest, bared from chin to belly-button. Note the rate, depth and rhythm of chest movements — more can be seen by standing 2m back than by peering closely. One side of the chest may move less well than the other in pneumonia or collapsed lung (pneumothorax). Look at the accessory muscles that strain when breathing is labored — flared nostrils, gasping mouth, taut neck muscles and indrawn intercostal muscles that lie between the ribs.

Feel: by placing hands lightly against the sides of his chest with fingers pointing towards his armpits. Unequal movement can be felt more easily on deep breathing. Percussion of the chest — thumping with one finger against a finger of the other hand placed against the chest — is hard to interpret even for a trained physician.

Listen: to both sides of the chest, front and back, from top to bottom, and have the victim breathe gently through his mouth. Air entry should be equal on both sides and can be noted by moving an ear from one side to the other. Breath sounds should be clear and unrestricted. Wheeze is easily picked up on expiration. Other sounds of fluid in the air passages may be heard as rough crackling like crumpling paper, or fine crackling like rubbing hair between fingers in front of the ear (crepitations). At high altitude think of pulmonary edema.

Asthma, bronchitis, and pneumonia may be difficult to distinguish.

ASTHMA

Asthma is associated with hay fever and eczema. It may be precipitated by acute infection, aspirin, specific allergens (pollens, dust), exertion, excitement and cold air. Spasm of the bronchi causes wheezing especially on expiration, a tight chest and dry cough which later produces sputum when infection is present. Feel the pulse racing and listen for crackles and expiratory wheeze with an ear on the back of the victim's chest.

Rx: salbutamol (D.8.1) puffer; if it does not settle, a course of dexamethasone (D.4.1). In a severe asthmatic attack, adrenaline (D.7.2).

Status Asthmaticus is an attack of asthma lasting more than 24 hours. The symptoms are as above together with shortness of breath and cyanosis. The victim becomes drowsy and can rapidly slide into shock and die.

Rx: salbutamol (D.8.1), dexamethasone (D.4.1).

BRONCHITIS

Infection of the upper respiratory tract, the common cold, laryngitis or pharyngitis, are all commonly caused by viruses and frequently develop a superimposed secondary bacterial infection. Wheeze, fever and cough with yellow or green spit are produced. Crackles can be heard at the back of the chest.

PNEUMONIA

Pneumonia may be bacterial or viral; it causes cough with rusty or bloody sputum, fever and rigors. Breathing is rapid and painful owing to pleurisy.

Act: Secretions; inhale steam from a kettle or billy-can of boiling water, which can also be poured onto a teaspoonful of tincture of benzoin put in an old tin. A towel over the head makes a tent in order to concentrate the steam, but beware of scalding. Sip a cup of boiling water adding one tablespoon each of baking soda and salt. Thump the chest with the person lying on alternating sides and head tipped down.

Rx: salbutamol (D.8.1), a bronchial relaxant, in a mild attack of bronchospasm.

codeine (D.1.3) at night dampens cough to allow sleep but should not be used by day. Expectorant cough mixtures are popular but their effect is not proven.

cephalosporin (D.2.1) or co-trimoxazole (D.2.2) antibiotic for at least 1 week if the sputum is yellow or green, or if there is a fever.

morphine (D.1.4) may be needed for severe pleuritic pain in order to allow full breathing, but be prepared to reverse with naloxone (D.1.5).

dexamethasone (D.4.1) i/v, or by mouth, should be used in people who have been on steroids before; it may help in asthma.

oxygen: relieves breathlessness and cyanosis.

ALLERGY

The body responds to the introduction of foreign substances (antigens) by forming protein antibodies in the blood. An excessive stimulus may cause an allergic (hypersensitivity) reaction owing to release of histamine. For example, some people are mildly sensitive to penicillin and break out in a rash; severe reactions result in life-threatening anaphylactic shock. Common allergies result from contact with pollens and moulds, house dust and house mites, animal dander and hair, and certain foods like shellfish and chocolate. The symptoms, uncomfortable but not dangerous, are of asthma, hay fever (with running nose and eyes), or hives on the skin with itchy raised weals.

Rx: antihistamine (D.3) allays itching and speeds the disappearance of symptoms.

ANAPHYLAXIS

Immediate, severe, shock-like and often fatal reactions follow contact with an antigen — a bee or wasp sting, a drug (especially penicillin and aspirin), injection of immune serum (tetanus antiserum and snake antivenin) or, rarely, of vaccines. The symptoms are of apprehension and shock, choking, wheezy asthma with cough and cyanosis. Blotchy skin weals develop all over the body; untreated, the victim may lose consciousness, convulse and die within 5 to 10 minutes.

People with known sensitivity to bee or wasp stings should carry a first aid kit with a preloaded syringe of adrenaline.

Rx: adrenaline 0.3 — 1.0ml if 1:1000 i/m or s/c repeated in the first 5 to 10 minutes. Keep open the victim's airway and place him in the draining position. Put up i/v fluids. [Hydrocortisone] 100-250mg i/v in the first 30 minutes followed by a course of dexamethasone orally.

Gut

INDIGESTION

Stomach gas may cause a bloated, dyspeptic feeling behind the lower end of the breast-bone (sternum), or in the upper abdomen (epigastrium); it is often relieved by a hearty belch. The discomfort, colloquially known as heart-burn, may be so severe as to mimic the chest pain of a heart attack and many people have spent the night in intensive care wired up to electronic monitors until cured by a glass of milk and a dose of antacid white medicine. Farting becomes a social problem, especially at high altitude.

One serious American wilderness medicine text gives the advice ". . . one should not attempt to ignite rectal gas or direct a stream of gas into a campfire. Backflashes and minor burns are a real risk".

Avoid heavy meals but do not let the stomach lie empty for long
periods because stomach acid starts to graw away at the lining,
which is how ulcers start. Every 2 hours eat a cookie with a glass
of milk, which coats the stomach and gives the natural
hydrochloric acid something to work on. Aspirin is very irritating,
and in a sensitive person one tablet may spark off a significant
bleed (hematemesis). Avoid fried food, fats, spices, nicotine,
coffee and alcohol, all of which stimulate gastric acid production.
What joys are there left in life?.

Rx: aluminium hydroxide (D.9.1), the base of a multitude of
antacids; the liquid gives quickest relief but tablets are more
convenient for the pocket and can be bought across the counter in
many proprietary forms.

Simple indigestion may be difficult to distinguish from acid
regurgitation, peptic ulcer and gall-bladder disease. In every
instance when far from help treat as above, and if the symptoms
persist seek a doctor for a proper diagnosis.

ACID REGURGITATION
The lining of the gullet (esophagus) does not take kindly to
stomach acid; regurgitating water-brash causes burning pain
behind the sterum. This also occurs when a portion of the upper
stomach slides through a gap in the diaphragm into the chest
(hiatus hernia). Discomfort is worst when lying flat and may cause
vomiting; it is relieved by sleeping propped-up, and taking the
precautions described above.

PEPTIC ULCER
Gastric or duodenal ulcers cause gnawing pain in the pit of the
stomach coming on a couple of hours after meals, and only
partially relieved by indigestion treatment. A history may reveal
that the ulcer has been lying dormant for years, but then may
flare up under stress or unaccustomed eating and living
conditions. The danger is of a sudden, torrential, life-threatening
bleed (hematemesis) or perforation (peritonitis).

Rx: antacids (D.9.1) and famotidine (D.9.2) for at least a
month even if symptoms subside.

GALL-BLADDER DISEASE
Mild gall-bladder inflammation (cholecystitis) causes indigestion

and constant pain under the right rib margin; it is also felt in the right shoulder tip and/or through to the back under the right shoulder blade. Jaundice, seen as yellow whites of the eyes and a tinge to the skin, may be present with pale, putty-like stools and mahogany-dark urine. Food is nauseating.

Rx: cephalosporin (D.2.1)

A severe gall-bladder attack owing to a gallstone lodged in the duct causes excruciating colic, the victim is very sick and needs urgent surgical help.

JAUNDICE

Infectious hepatitis is the most likely cause of jaundice in travelers. The victim feels rotten for about a week before the whites of the eyes turn yellow and the skin begins to itch, eventually going yellow. Pain is usually absent. He may feel better once jaundice appears. Full recovery may take months and be prolonged if rest, which is the only treatment, is curtailed.

Several infectious diseases, especially those caused by viruses, have a similar prodrome of malaise before the illness becomes manifest, for example, influenza and glandular fever (mononucleosis).

CONSTIPATION

Not drinking enough is the commonest cause of this misery. Dehydrated foods make it worse and contribute to noisome gas. Eat a preventive diet of bran, cereal roughage, and fruit. If this fails use a laxative, mineral oil, bisacodyl (D.9.4) or a soap and water enema, in that order. Dehydration can turn the stools to concrete and ruin a trip (and may even require manual removal with a well-greased finger).

DIARRHEA (see p.227)

VOMITING

A stomach upset from dietary indiscretion or food poisoning may cause a short burst of vomiting, which usually settles in a day by stopping eating and taking sips of fluid only. If vomiting persists suspect some more serious intra-abdominal mischief and seek medical help.

Skin Problems

ECZEMA (dermatitis): associated with allergies and contact with certain drugs, nickel and cosmetics.
 Rx: betamethasone (D.11.1) ointment.

IMPETIGO: a superficial infection of the skin usually with staphylococcus. A vesicle becomes a pustule that forms characteristic yellow crusty scabs usually on the face.
 Rx: cephalosporin (D.2.1) by mouth.

TINEA: a fungal infection causing athlete's foot and dhobie itch of the crotch manifest an irritating, red, silver-scaly rash.
 Rx: clotrimazole (D.11.2) antifungal cream.

SCABIES: the mite thrives in bedding and unclean clothing. It burrows forming a pin-head vesicle, which becomes scratched because it is maddeningly irritating especially when warm in bed.
 Rx: [benzyl benzoate] applied from neck to toes, and repeated in 5 days.

LICE & NITS: lay eggs on hair shafts.
 Rx: [benzyl benzoate.]

Psychological problems

Many psychological problems are alleviated by the peace of the wilderness. For this very reason many of us choose it as our escape from worldly cares. However when anxiety is manifest we must be able to distinguish panic from psychosis.

PANIC
Under arduous conditions or during a difficult wilderness journey a person may loose his nerve and become frightened, agitated and acutely anxious. Although rational, he is paralysed with fear and becomes ineffective.
 Act: talk to the person with calm reassurance; anger will only provoke him. If still out of control when back at camp, Rx: lorazepam (D.5.1). Wait until next morning to see if he returns to

normal after a good sleep; if he does, the condition is panic and not psychosis, which would take much longer to settle. The person will probably be deeply ashamed of the episode, so encourage him to talk and get it off his chest. Such emotions might be the lot of any of us on another occasion so empathy is needed.

PSYCHOSIS (madness)

Madness, as distinct from panic, does not usually start out of the blue without some previous warning of mental imbalance. In selecting wilderness companions be wary of someone with a record of strange behavior; your intuitive feelings may be right. The person may loose touch with reality and have bizarre hallucinations. He feels that other people are ganging up on him, and he may appear so convincing that you begin to wonder who is crazy, you or he. He tends to over-react to normal situations and may be violent and excited, or passive and withdrawn. Once the acute phase of a psychotic episode has passed, a more drawn-out depression sets in when the person is most likely to attempt suicide.

Rx: lorazepam (D.5.1) will sedate the person; if he becomes violent try to prevent him from injuring himself and others. Forcible restraint may only worsen the situation making him more excited, but may be needed in the last resort.

15 EYES

The eyeball horrifies and few people can even bring themselves to inspect it closely. Only careful looking, preferably with magnification, will allow intelligent treatment.

Ask: the person to read newsprint of various sizes from normal reading distance, with glasses if he usually wears them, and using each eye separately. Was each eye perfect before the present problem arose? Recording the vision now will help in following progress. Is the eye painful? Scratches of the window of the eye (cornea) commonly give the sensation of a foreign body; infection of the conjunctiva (the thin, loose, transparent membrane over the white sclera of the eye) feels like grit or sand in the eyes. Are there persistent flashes of light, blurred patches in the vision, or strange visual sensations? All are abnormal.

Look: at the eye with a flashlight and a magnifying glass, a loupe or a camera lens. A drop of local anesthetic proparacaine (D.12.4) placed in the gutter of the lid (fornix) makes the task easier because the person will relax his tightly screwed up eyes; it takes less than a minute to act.

Lids — pull down the lower lid to look for a foreign body in the fornix; Then evert the upper lid as this is a common place for uninvited matter to lodge. When anesthetized sweep a match-stick, with cotton wool wound onto the tip, along both upper and lower fornices. If nothing appears leave some eye ointment in the lower fornix and a foreign body may eventually float out.

Lashes — inturned lashes scratch the cornea like barbs and are the source of much discomfort. Pluck them out with tweezers.

Conjunctiva — red and swollen conjunctiva denotes inflammation or infection, which causes aversion to bright light, tearing and yellow discharge.

Cornea — is normally clear and shiny. If fluorescein dye from a dampened impregnated paper strip is touched against the inner

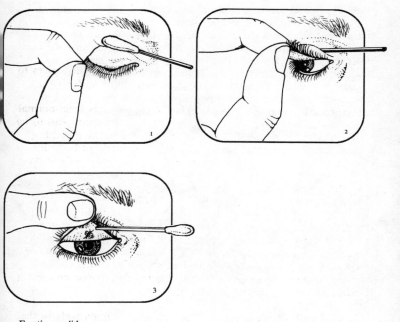

Everting eyelid

aspect of the lower lid, any breach in the corneal surface caused by abrasions, ulcers or foreign bodies shows up as a bright-green stain.

Pupil — is normally circular and constricts when light is shone into it; an eccentric pupil suggests problems in the anterior chamber of the eye.

Act: dark glasses or a pirate's patch keep out light, which is painful. A firm bandage over several eye pads gives pressure on the lids and stops blinking, which irritates the cornea. An eye pad held on with sticky tape alone does not provide enough pressure to keep the lids closed and becomes loose, damp and uncomfortable.

Rx: *tea*; contains tannic acid which is astringent, soothing, cheap, available and there is no limit to how often it can be instilled. For an uncomfortable, scratchy, painful eye squeeze cold tea from a moist tea bag (Darjeeling or Earl Grey are equally effective) into the lower fornix. If there is infection with pussy discharge use chloramphenicol (D.12.1), but antibiotics are much over-prescribed; they all have chemical bases, which sting and cause irritation that can compound an existing problem.

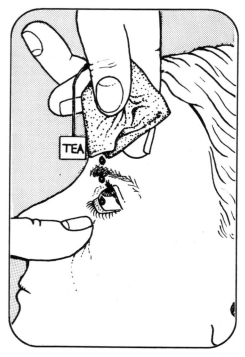

Eye drops

Local anesthetic: proparacaine (D.12.4) "freezes" the eye allowing foreign bodies to be removed. Cover the eye afterwards until sensation returns. Local anesthetic delays healing so must not be used over a long period to relieve pain, but it could be life-saving in allowing a snow-blind person to return to a lower camp.

Pupil dilator: homatropine 2% (D.12.3) mydriatic twice daily; dilates the pupil and relieves painful spasm that follows abrasion or injury of the cornea; it blurs vision making the eye sensitive to light, so use dark glasses or a patch. Homatropine lasts for 24 hours after the last drop, unlike atropine which dilates the pupil for a couple of weeks. The remote chance of inducing glaucoma should not discourage the use of a short-acting mydriatic; besides relieving pain it also offers a better view of the back of the eye for someone with the skill to use an ophthalmoscope. However, it should not be used in the presence of a head injury because it confuses the pupil signs of cerebral compression, or in hyphema when blood cells may block the drainage angle and cause glaucoma.

Antibiotic: chloramphenicol (D.12.1); use antibiotics when there is danger of infection, an ulcer or if pus is present. Ointment stays around the eye and need only be put in twice a day, but it feels gooey and fogs the vision; drops must be instilled at least 6 hourly.

Steroid: dexamethasone (D.12.2) steroid; has a magical effect on many red eyes but should be avoided unless in skilled hands because it delays healing, and if used in herpes virus infection may rot the cornea.

Infection and inflammation — painful red eye(s)

INFECTION
Conjunctivitis — usually both eyes feel gritty as though sand is in them; they look red, may water and discharge, and they resent bright light (photophobia). The vision is unaffected.
  Rx: antibiotic (D.12.1), dark glasses.

Corneal ulcer — fluorescein shows up a stain, usually central and circular. Vision will be interrupted if the ulcer lies on the visual axis in the center of the cornea. Corneal ulcers are usually caused by bacteria, may take 1-2 weeks to heal, and can scar permanently.

Rx: mydriatic (D.12.3), antibiotic (D.12.1), dark glasses.

Herpes Simplex — a mature herpetic corneal ulcer has squiggly, branching arms (dendrites) that stain with fluorescein. Look for "kissing", or "cold" sores on the lips which give away the diagnosis. Herpes is a virus, hard to diagnose without magnification and difficult to treat. If someone has had herpes infection before and gets a red eye presume it is herpes again.

Rx: mydriatic (D.12.3), [arabinase (Viroptic)] 2 hourly for 3 days, then 6 hourly for a week.

INFLAMMATION

Iritis — usually a single eye becomes red, painful, photophobic and the vision is blurred. The pupil may be stuck to the lens; it appears irregular and is immobile in response to light. Iritis is difficult to diagnose without huge magnification. A history of previous attacks should arouse suspicion.

. Rx: mydriatic (D.12.3), steroid (D.12.2), dark glasses.

Contact lens keratitis — contact lenses may scratch the cornea causing painful inflammation. If the lens is left out the cornea usually heals in 24 to 48 hours. Tea will soothe meanwhile. To remove a soft contact lens, moisten the tip of the finger, hold the lids open with the other hand, look down, and pinch it off with finger and thumb.

Eyelid cysts and styes — occur as uncomfortable, red, swollen lumps on the lid margins, sometimes with a core of pus.

Act: try to pull out any lash that may appear to arise from the center of the lump. Apply heat by winding cloth round a wooden stick, dipping it in boiling water and holding it as close to the eye as possible without scalding the lid. The heat will soothe and the cyst or stye may come to a head and burst. Antibiotics locally are to no avail.

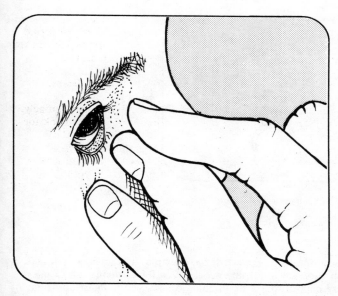

Removing contact lens

Injuries

CLOSED INJURY (non-penetrating)
Subconjunctival hemorrhage — a mild bang on the eye, or even rubbing it during sleep, can spill a single drop of blood that spreads out under the loose sheet of conjunctiva. The eye goes a horrifying scarlet, will change through all the colors of the rainbow and fade within three weeks. It is of no sinister import provided the posterior limit of the blood is visible by turning the eye towards the nose; if in a serious injury with bruised and black eyes, no posterior limit is visible, suspect bleeding from the brain — a very serious sign.

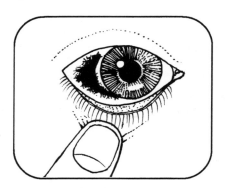

Eye injury: subconjunctival hemorrhage

Corneal abrasion — caused, for example, by inturned eyelashes, a brush with a twig or pine needle, or a flying wood chip. The eye is very painful for 24 to 48 hours by which time most abrasions are healed; if pain persists more than 2 days consider an ulcer or infection.

Act: pluck out an inturned lash for instant relief. If the cause is otherwise, use tea.

Rx: mydriatic (D.12.3), antibiotic (D.12.1), analgesic (D.1), dark glasses, if infection is suspected.

Foreign body — a speck of dirt or metal embedded in the cornea can often be seen with the naked eye. Sometimes it is lodged in the fornix of the upper or lower lid, or is stuck to the underside of the upper lid where it scratches with every blink.

Act: lie the person down to avoid fainting; then wash the eye with copious water.

Rx: local anesthetic (D.12.4) 2 drops. Try to wipe the speck away with a folded corner of tissue. If it won't budge use a pushing motion with the end of a matchstick approaching cautiously from the side to avoid digging into the cornea.

Rx: mydriatic, tea; only use antibiotic if infection is evident.

Even if a metal foreign body is removed residual iron pigment
will form subsequently a ring of rust where the metal lay in
contact with the cornea. A rust ring must be removed later by an
eye specialist. Observe for perforation (see below).

BURNS
When the face is burned the lids take the brunt of the damage
because blinking usually occurs before flame touches the cornea.
Corneal burns may be caused by fire sparks, ultra-violet light and
chemicals.

Ultra-violet burn (Snow Blindness). Sun reflects strongly off snow
and light-colored rocks; its rays penetrate hazy cloud and become
more powerful with altitude. The resulting ultra-violet burn of the
cornea causes intensely painful inflammation so the eyes are
screwed up tightly. About six hours after burning swelling of the
conjunctiva and blistering of the cornea prevent the victim from
seeing out, he becomes temporarily "blind" and has to be led or

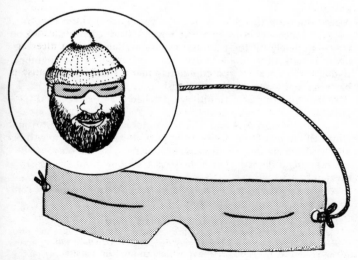

Snow goggles

carried to a lower camp, with all the attendant risks.

Act: wear goggles or dark glasses with side-shields to exclude glare. In emergency cut horizontal slits in a piece of cardboard or duct-tape doubled on itself, and tie it round the head with a piece of string, like Inuit snow-goggles.

Rx: analgesics (D.1) and tea; local anesthetic drops (D.12.4) will relieve pain and spasm long enough for the victim to reach camp unaided and so may be life-saving. Do not use anesthetic drops for prolonged pain relief afterwards. After reaching safety both eyes are then treated like severe corneal abrasions.

Chemical burns — caused by battery acid, or lime.

Act: wash the eye immediately and repeatedly with copious water for at least 5 minutes, and remove any lumps of chemical. Wash with bicarbonate of soda (baking soda) for acid burns, which usually heal quickly; milk or vinegar for alkali burns the consequences of which are often severe.

Rx: mydriatic (D.12.3), analgesic (D.1)

BRUISING

After a blow on the globe of the eye the injury is commonly in the *anterior chamber*, in front of the pupil, called a hyphema. Blood may completely fill the chamber so vision is obscured. After a few hours it settles forming a crescent at the bottom of the chamber. If the victim does not rest completely there is danger of more bleeding and a serious threat to vision.

Act: complete rest with one eye patched for 4 to 5 days if possible.

Rx: analgesics (D.1) and a sedative, lorazepam (D.5.1), to make lying still easier. Do not dilate the pupil because blood may block off the drainage angle and cause glaucoma. Use tea only. If the eye remains inflamed after 4 days start steroid drops (D.12.2) every 6 hours.

Alternatively, the injury may be in the *posterior chamber*; (only visible with an ophthalmoscope).

Bleeding into the vitreous jelly; vision is very blurred and no red background is visible with an ophthalmoscope, just a black reflection.
Retinal detachment; a shadow may appear like a curtain falling across the vision, wavy shadows of matter float around in the vitreous, and there may be a sensation of flashing lights.

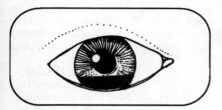

Eye injury: hyphaema

Act: both conditions urgently need an eye surgeon. Patch the eye meanwhile and rest as much as possible.

High Altitude Retinal Hemorrhage (HARH); (see page 215)

OPEN INJURY (penetrating)

Infection and disorganization of the interior of the eye are hazards of penetrating injury. A wound may be seen across the cornea (less commonly the white sclera) but often the wound is tiny and seals over disguising the mischief. Vision is reduced and the eye is red. The iris lies close against the back of the cornea. The pupil may be irregular and pear-shaped because part of the iris gets caught in the wound. To test for anterior chamber fluid touch a fluorescein paper strip on the upper part of the eye and observe closely for a streak of fluorescence dribbling down where eye fluid and dye mix.

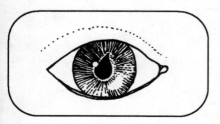

Eye injury: pear shaped pupil

Act: penetrating injuries are very serious and warrant an eye surgeon's urgent attention. Sympathetic inflammation can occur within 2 weeks in the opposite uninjured eye leading to blindness.

Rx: double dose of antibiotic cephalosporin (D.2.1) by mouth, analgesics (D.1), dark glasses.

EYELID INJURY

Always check the globe of the eye for associated injury. Eyelid repair requires great surgical skill in order to restore accurately the windscreen-wiper mechanism. Beware an injury in the corner of the eye near the nose where the tiny tear ducts may have been torn; they need speedy repair.

Rx: antibiotic drops (D. 12.1), pain-killers, and patch meanwhile.

FACIAL FRACTURE

The bony ring around the orbit may be disrupted so the eyeball sinks causing double vision (diplopia). The cheek is flattened and tender, and sometimes a step may be felt in the smooth lower rim of the orbit by running a finger along it.

Act: a pirate's patch eliminates diplopia until a surgeon can be reached.

ACUTE MIDDLE-EAR INFECTION (otitis media)

Searing pain develops in the affected ear, usually with high fever. Hearing is dulled. Fluid under pressure in the middle-ear may result in rupture of the ear-drum and discharge of clear fluid. Earache may also be caused by a faulty upper wisdom tooth.

Act: a light cotton-wool plug in the outer-ear keeps out cold, which aggravates pain. Warm olive oil dropped into the ear and placing the ear against a hot-water-bottle, is soothing.

Rx: cephalosporin (D.2.1) by mouth.

FOREIGN BODY

Small round objects and insects may lodge in the outer-ear. Wax is wafted towards the outside by hairs in the ear canal.

Act: pull back the earlobe in order to straighten the canal and to give a clear view in as far as the drum. Lubricate the ear passage with a couple of drops of liquid paraffin or cooking olive oil. Turn the head on one side and shake vigorously. Gently flush the ear with clean, warm water using a syringe; 5 to 10 irrigations should allow the foreign matter to slide out. Do not dig for wax or poke around with match-sticks because the ear drum may be damaged. If a foreign body is seen in the canal try to pick it out with tweezers or a wire loop maneuvered past it and then withdrawn.

EUSTACHEAN TUBE BLOCKAGE

When the tube leading from the back of the throat to the middle-ear is blocked by swelling owing to a throat infection, or by sudden change in pressure such as altitude change in airplanes, hearing is dulled and the person feels like yawning to relieve the block.

Act: yawn, swallow hard or blow out against a closed nose, mouth and throat. Blockage usually clears in its own time. If it is imperative to fly when suffering from a cold, chew gum before take-off and landing.

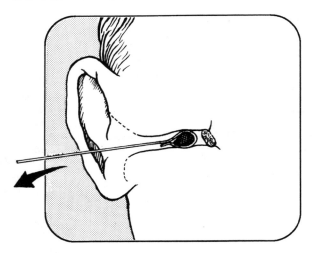

Foreign body in ear

Rx: ephedrine (D.14.1) decongestant nose drops and steam inhalation every 6 hours.

LABRYINTHITIS
Virus infection in the middle-ear may follow a cold; it upsets the balance so the person feels unsteady, nauseated and utterly miserable.

Rx: antihistamine (D.3) helps a little but is sedative, which may be an asset while resting. Time is the healer but it may take 6 weeks.

MENIERE'S DISEASE
Severe vertigo induces falling to the ground, nausea, vomiting, and profuse sweating, followed by deafness and ringing in the ears — a most unpleasant combination. Reassure the person it will pass, and restrict salt.

Rx: antihistamines (D.3)

Mouth

MOUTH ULCERS

Canker sores — are painful and irritating.
Traumatic ulcers — a tooth rubs an ulcer on the inside of the cheek.

Act: mouth washes of salt or baking soda. Gentian violet paint made from crystals is mucky to use but heals mucosal surfaces.

Herpes simplex — Sores frequently accompany colds. They are contagious and occur on the lips, inside the nostrils, and rarely though much publicized, on the genitals. They form blisters which crust, scab and heal after 2 to 3 weeks.

Act: keep the blisters dry by dabbing with alcohol; refrain from kissing. Wash all eating utensils and cups carefully.

Nose

COMMON COLD

Colds are caused by viruses but are a common nuisance. Runny nose, sore throat and fever usually clear within a week. Antibiotics have no effect on viruses and should not be used.

Act: avoid contagion by sleeping head-to-toe in a well-ventilated tent. Use steam inhalation with tincture of benzoin, gargle with 1 tsp of salt in 1 liter of water. Garlic cloves, chili peppers, mustard plasters, or horse radish may help; give zinc tablets a try but don't waste money, space or energy carrying extra vitamins.

Rx: paracetamol (D.1.1), ephedrine (D.14.1) nose drops, antibiotic (D.2.) if a cold on the chest leads to bronchitis with yellow or green spit that indicates pus from a secondary bacterial infection.

SINUSITIS

Infection of the air sinuses around the face produces yellow or green snot. Severe headache is felt over the forehead or behind the eyes, and pain and tenderness are felt over the cheek or brow overlying the sinuses, or in the upper teeth. Frontal sinusitis rarely may spread back to the brain causing meningitis.

Act: inhale steam in order to encourage drainage by liquefying

snot, and shrinking the swollen mucosal lining of the air passages.
   Rx: decongestants (D.14.1), antibiotics (D.2).

HAY FEVER (allergic rhinitis)
Watery nasal discharge, itchy eyes and nose, sneezing, are signs of
nasal congestion.
   Rx: decongestant (D.14.1), antihistamine (D.3).

NOSEBLEED (epistaxis)
Bleeding usually stops after a few minutes with ice and pressure
alone, but occasionally it may be so uncontrollable as to threaten
life. Bleeding is never a safety-valve, as folklore would have it, but
it may indicate high blood pressure. Bleeding arises from the
septum between the nostrils or high in the nose, well out of sight.
   Act: sit the person leaning slightly forward with the head
bowed. Encourage him to blow out of his nostrils clots, which do
nothing to stop further bleeding and just dam up behind them
blood that trickles down the back of the throat into the stomach
and will make him vomit. Identify from which side the blood is
coming. Place a cold compress, preferably of ice or snow wrapped
in a damp cloth, across the bridge of the nose. Squeeze the
nostrils for 20 minutes below where the bone and soft nose
cartilage join. Discourage breathing through the nose, picking at
clots, blowing the nose, or sneezing, for 24 hours. If the air is
very dry, as at altitude or in severe cold, apply vaseline to the
affected side once the bleeding has stopped.

   If bleeding persists push a gauze pack soaked in adrenaline (D.7.2) or
   ephedrine (D.14.1) as high as possible up the offending nostril and
   leave it there for 24 to 48 hours. If re-bleeding starts on removing the
   gauze, re-pack the nostril. The wilderness is no place for the amateur to
   try packing the post-nasal space via the mouth — a maneuver fraught
   with hazard.
      Packing the post-nasal space should only be done by someone with
   the appropriate skill. Sew 3 long strings of thread securely through a
   rolled gauze square. Pass a soft rubber catheter (or a Foley catheter,
   and blow up the balloon later) through the bleeding nostril, past the
   pharynx and out through the mouth. Tie 2 of the strings to the catheter
   tip and draw them back through the nose. Guide the pack up behind
   the uvula while pulling on the strings. Anchor the strings by tying them
   over a rolled gauze up against the nostril. Pull the third string out of

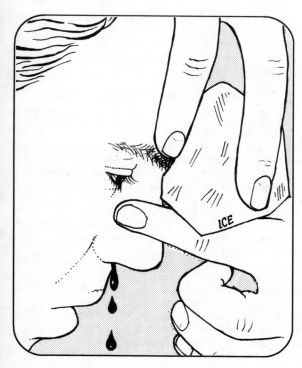

Stopping nosebleed

the mouth and tape it to the face in order to pull on later in order to remove the pack.

Leave the pack in not longer than 4 days.

BROKEN NOSE

An isolated fracture and the associated black eyes mar beauty; if associated with other facial fractures the injury is more significant and means a serious head injury.

Act: ice reduces the swelling until a surgeon can deal with the fracture.

Throat

SORE THROAT
Virus infection, the commonest form of sore throat, looks fiery
red, there is no pus, and the infection does not respond to
antibiotics.

Act: gargle with warm salt water and suck throat lozenges.

HIGH ALTITUDE RAW THROAT
Breathing cold, dry air at high altitude is the cause.

Act: moisten the air by inhaling steam from a bowl, or sniff a
billycan on the stove while making a tea brew, but don't scald
your nose or throat. Expeditions never carry enough lozenges; if
short, suck on hard candies and drink lots of fluid.

TONSILLITIS OR STREP THROAT
Yellow flecks of pus lie on the red, swollen tonsils; glands under
the angle of the jaw swell and swallowing hurts.

Rx: cephalosporin (D.2.1), salt-water gargles.

QUINSY
An abscess develops in the region of the tonsil bed, the soft palate
swells and swallowing may become almost impossible.

Act: if medical help is far off, urgent, decisive lancing with a
sterile blade into the most swollen part of the affected tonsil
releases a gush of pus, but this may be very difficult if the jaw is
shut tight in spasm (trismus). Then gargle with warm salt water.

Rx: cephalosporin (D.2.1).

GLANDULAR FEVER (infectious mononucleosis)
The victim feels rotten, sluggish and washed-out for no apparent
reason. A thick yellow slough in the sore throat looks far worse
than it feels. Lymph glands in the neck, armpit and groin swell.

Act: rest is essential (ideally for 4 weeks) because the disease
can recur with activity; rarely an enlarged spleen can rupture. It
may take several months before the person feels full of vigor
again.

Rx: dexamethasone (D.4.1) if the throat swells so that
swallowing and breathing are impaired.

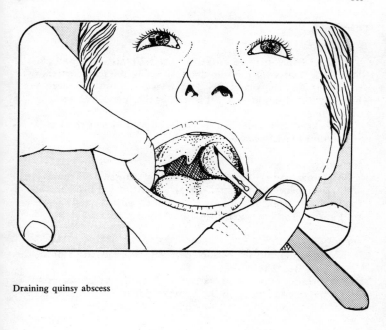

Draining quinsy abscess

SWALLOWED FOREIGN BODY
Fish-bones stuck in the gullet may be dislodged, and carried
onwards, by eating dry bread. An immovable chicken bone will
have to be taken to a surgeon. A piece of meat stuck in the gullet
may threaten life — the Heimlich maneuver (see p. 59) may
dislodge it.

Rarely emergency cricothyrotomy is needed.

Face and jaws

FRACTURE

The facial bones may be broken in several places in a bad smash. Suspect a fracture if the bite does not bring the teeth together normally, or if the victim has double vision, a bruised cheek, a black eye, and if you can feel a step in the line of his lower eye socket bone.

Act: expert treatment is needed. Feed a fluid diet through a straw until the jaw can be fixed.

DISLOCATION

Rx: lorazepam (D.5.1) to relax the jaw, support the lower jaw with the fingers of both hands, place your thumbs over his molars (padded to prevent him biting them), then push steadily down and backwards. The jaw should slide back into place.

HICCOUGH

This distressing and unpleasant rhythmic reflex contraction of the diaphragm needs to be interrupted.

Act: drink a cup of iced water fast; hold the breath or breathe into a paper bag; press on the eyeballs, or tickle the back of the throat with a feather — all to stimulate the vagus nerve.

Teeth

TOOTHACHE

Toothache can be so disabling as to render a person useless, therefore prevent it by having a careful dental check before setting off on an expedition, eating a diet with adequate vitamin C, and cleaning the teeth regularly. In the absence of a toothbrush rub the teeth with a wet finger covered with salt or baking soda, or with a peeled green stick. Chewing gum cleans the mouth and exercises the gums.

Intense hot or cold makes diseased or exposed teeth painful. Cold teeth may fracture suddenly when warmed by a hot drink or biting on hard food. Dental pain comes under legion disguises, aching, throbbing, searing, and it may be difficult to localize to a particular tooth especially in the early stages. Pain often affects

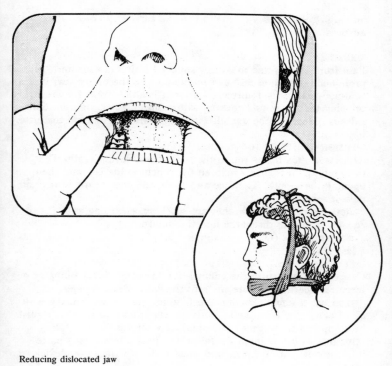

Reducing dislocated jaw

adjacent teeth and may spread from the upper to the lower jaw and vice-versa, but never across the mid-line. An amateur in the field can give only simple treatment in order to tide the victim over until he can see a proper dentist.

FINDING AN ACHING TOOTH
Tap the suspected tooth gently on the top and side with a metal instrument, preferably a blunt dental probe. A diseased tooth will hurt. Do not stick the point into the exposed cavity or into the softened exposed root. Cold and heat worsen pain in living teeth,

although cold relieves discomfort in the early stage of a tooth abscess.

SINUSITIS
Pain from an infected maxillary sinus (the air space behind the prominence of the cheek) can mimic pain in the upper jaw; it is a common reason for faulty extraction of healthy teeth. In sinusitis pressing the cheek or knocking with a finger hurts; pain on both sides is unlikely to be dental. Pussy snot discharges from the nose.

COMMON CAUSES OF TOOTHACHE
Abscess — Pus forms round the root of a decaying tooth. The throbbing pain is partly relieved by clenching the jaw and then opening the mouth. The face and jaw swell, the breath stinks and pain is severe.

Act: hot salt mouth-washes are soothing, cleansing and encourage pus to discharge into the mouth.

Rx: antibiotic (D.2.1), analgesic (D.1); extract the tooth only as a last resort.

Cavity — A breach in the enamel due to decay, a lost filling or a fractured tooth, lays bare the sensitive inner dentine layer.

Act: use a temporary dressing of zinc oxide powder mixed with oil of cloves, or a synthetic tooth cement from a tube (which must be stoppered to prevent hardening). Do not dig out any filling remnants with a pointed dental probe. Push the dressing paste into the hole with a finger and press it down with a matchstick.

Exposed tooth root — When open to the cold exposed roots cause pain which may develop into chronic toothache if left unattended.

Act: avoid heavy brushing and contact with very hot or cold.

INFECTIONS
Bacterial (Vincent's infection, trench mouth) — Poor oral hygiene allows plaques to grow next to the gums which become infected. The gums may swell painfully, bleed and ulcerate causing an evil odor.

Act: use a toothbrush carefully. Gentian violet paint, made up from crystals, though messy to use, deals with most mouth ulcers.

Rx: antibiotics (D.2).

Pericoronitis — Food debris collects under the gum flap over a partially-erupted 3rd molar tooth. Infection starts, the gums swell and are further traumatized when pinched in chewing. Soon the person is unable to chew and the mouth is foul and painful.

Act: vigorous rinsing with hot salt-water. If possible use a bent hypodermic needle to reach under the flap into the crevices of the gum and flush out pus and debris with salt water.

Rx: antibiotics (D.2).

DISLOCATED OR AVULSED TEETH
Use warm salt mouthwash, replace the tooth immediately in the socket and try to stabilize it. It may 'take' like a free-graft.

TOOTH EXTRACTION
If far from help it may be best to extract a very painful tooth and allow the person, who would otherwise be an invalid, to continue with the expedition. If closer to help take out a tooth only as a last resort because skilful dentists can renovate some awful looking teeth. The art of extracting a loose or a bad tooth can be learned easily enough, but to remove a strong, live tooth is very difficult. You need the proper tools, preferably some local anesthetic, and a stoical patient. Lessons on how to inject local anesthetic should be taken from a dental surgeon before leaving on an expedition.

Rx: antibiotic (D.2) before attempting extraction; local anesthetic xylocaine 2% (D.17.1) with adrenalin 2ml for each tooth. This may not be effective if swelling is severe.

Upper jaw — Insert the needle just through the skin where the gum and the cheek join, near the apex of the affected tooth. Put in a few drops to start freezing; after 2 minutes advance the needle and distribute the remainder of the 2ml around the tooth. Do the same on the palate side where there will be more resistance because of tight tissues.

Lower jaw — Local anesthetic placed as described above may be effective from the premolars forward. Behind the molars a mandibular block is needed and this requires skill.

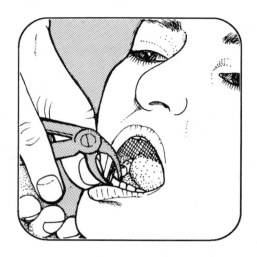

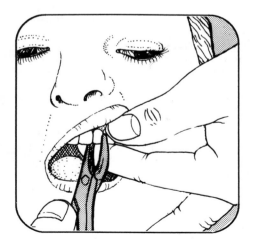

Lower and upper dental forceps

When the tooth is anesthetized, or the patient is sufficiently drugged to allow the ordeal, grasp the tooth with a pair of upper or lower dental forceps. Push the beaks of the forceps down each side of the tooth below the gum margin in order to get a hold as far down the root as possible. Use a sideways rocking and rotating movement to work the tooth loose. A disturbing crunch comes from the jaw as the roots separate from the socket. If the tooth breaks try to remove the remaining fragments but do not dig deeply for them or the socket may bleed profusely. Pinch the gums together to stop bleeding and have the victim bite on a damp gauze pack or paper tissue for 15 minutes. If it still will not stop pack the socket with gauze. Even removing the tooth crown alone may diminish the pain by letting pus discharge down the roots into the mouth. Smoking may restart the bleeding so desist for a day. Start hot salt mouth-washes on the second day.

17 HYPOTHERMIA

Hypothermia is generalized body chilling; local freezing is frostbite. Immersion injury occurs in the absence of freezing. Both hypothermia and frostbite may co-exist but hypothermia takes precedence in treatment because it can be fatal. Hypothermia is worsened by wet-cold, exhaustion, anxiety, injury, drugs and alcohol. Wet and wind are a lethal pair that chill a person more than dry-cold.

Denizens of polar climates and high altitudes, aware of the dangers of cold, dress in warm protective clothing. Inuit, Tibetans, Andean Indians and barefoot Himalayan hillmen survive intuitively in their hostile environment and appear to adapt to cold. But, all these people can suffer the ravages of cold like the rest of us unless they practice commonsense prevention.

Prevention

Plan carefully even the shortest outdoor expedition, watch for early signs of hypothermia and act promptly to avert it. Gauge the day's activity to the party's weakest member. Distance and speed of travel vary with terrain, weather, and load; walking too far too fast, carrying too heavy a load, and being cold, exhausted, hungry and demoralized, are the corner-stones of hypothermia. If the weather changes be prepared to abandon the original plan and take an easier, shorter route home. The measure of a good outdoorsman is knowing when to turn around.

Children and adolescents withstand cold less well than adults because their surface area is large in proportion to their weight, and generally they carry less subcutaneous fat. With less experience and smaller reserves of stamina and mental fiber, they tend to flag and give up hope unless strongly led. Women, by reason of their subcutaneous fat, are better insulated than men; but their smaller surface area and lower body weight cancel out this advantage.

Temperature control

The temperature of the central body core, which houses the vital organs (brain, heart, lungs, kidneys), is preserved at the expense of the surrounding shell (muscles, subcutaneous fat, skin). A temperature-regulating center in the brain senses changes in the temperature of blood flowing through it, and maintains a balance between heat gain and heat loss. Hypothermia occurs when more heat is lost than is produced.

A rise or fall in core temperature of 2°C causes noticeable symptoms; a drop of more than 6° to 7°C can kill. Core temperature is measured with a special low-reading thermometer below 35°C (95°F), placed in the rectum — an awkward maneuver in someone fully dressed. Mouth and armpit temperatures are initially inaccurate but never read less than true core temperature.

CONSERVING BODY HEAT

Insulation — Air and fat are poor conductors and therefore good insulators. Animals, when cold, raise their fur in order to trap air; likewise humans get goose-bumps. Wool, polypropylene and pile partially insulate by trapping air in the interstices of the fibers, which do not collapse when wet as does goose or eider down. The more layers of clothing the better the insulation. Water is an excellent conductor and thereby destroys insulation. The early Everest climbers at over 28,000ft were dressed in Norfolk tweed jackets and breeches dipped in water-repelling alum, several layers of Shetland-wool pullovers and long wool stockings.

Windproof, waterproof fabrics prevent entrapped, insulating air being displaced, and also diminish convection, conduction and evaporation. Breathable fabrics like Gore-Tex allow some ventilation; coated nylon does not, so water condenses on the inside of an outer garment and soaks the clothing underneath. Cotton jeans protect poorly against cold and wet. Sitting on a mattress or a pack provides insulation from the cold ground.

Blood vessel constriction — In the cold, automatic reflex control causes smooth muscle in blood vessels of the body shell to constrict and thus keep warm blood circulating in the core, preventing heat loss from the shell. The head, armpits and groins

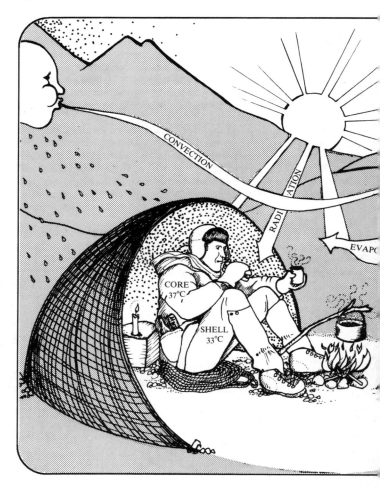

Heat gain and loss

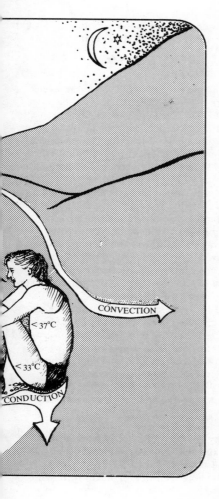

are areas of high heat loss because large blood vessels run through areas where the body wall is thin; therefore these areas need special protection when cold.

BODY HEAT LOSS

Convection — Wind speed determines the chill felt at an even temperature; air temperature alone is meaningless as a physiological measure of cold. On a windless, sunny day at $-40°C$ ($-40°F$) you can walk about lightly clad owing to solar radiation, but the least puff of wind will send you scurrying for shelter. At $0°C$ ($32°F$) with a 65kph (40mph) wind, cold may be intolerable. Wet-cold feels much chillier than dry-cold because conduction and evaporation are increased. Wind destroys air insulation by displacing trapped air, energy is expended in battling the wind, and evaporation is increased by wind blowing on a wet surface. The wind-chill index is a graphic plot of wind speed against temperature. Wind-chill applies only to exposed skin and is virtually irrelevant to clothed persons unless the clothing allows wind to penetrate. It can give the wrong message to people, for example victims of boating accidents, who are better out of the water clinging to the bottom of the boat than staying in the water and losing twenty times the heat by water conduction.

Convection also continues in the absence of wind because air next to the skin is warmed and rises away from the body. Heat is lost quickly from an uncovered head — so when your feet are cold put on a hat. Wear a wool scarf, make a snug fit at the wrists with Velcro or elastic, and tuck trousers into socks or use gaiters. Mittens allow fingers to warm each other by mutual contact whereas gloves isolate each digit. Silk gloves allow delicate touch, for example when handling a camera, and can be worn inside mittens.

Conduction — Heat flows by conduction directly from a warm body to wet clothes and to the cold ground. Wind and wet reduce insulation of clothing to one tenth of normal. During glacial stream crossings always wear long trousers for warmth, boots for sure footing, and belay securely with a rope. Legs immersed to the thigh cool fast; they move slower and slower and may finally collapse leading to drowning.

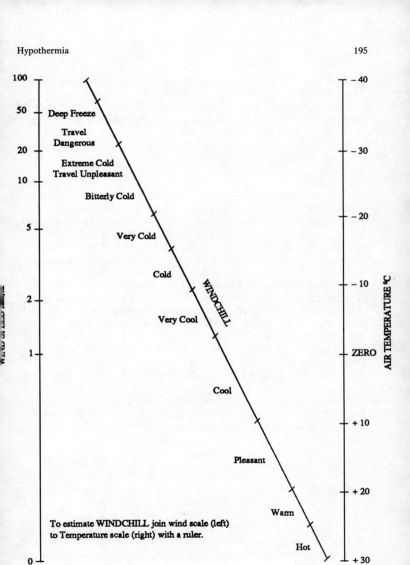

To estimate WINDCHILL join wind scale (left)
to Temperature scale (right) with a ruler.

Wind-chill index

Evaporation — To evaporate 1g of water requires 540 calories of heat. Body evaporation is caused by:

Sweating: 0.5l (1 pint) of fluid is normally lost daily through the skin, much more in hot climates and in dry-cold. During heavy exercise up to 1l may be lost each hour.

Breathing: warm breath condenses in cold air and breathing cold air cools the airway. Much water can be lost during heavy breathing.

Blood vessel dilatation — Alcohol dilates blood vessels causing warm blood to flow away from the core to the periphery. Drunks found dead in snow banks sometimes have thrown off their clothes because a flush of warm blood suffuses the body after the sympathetic nervous system finally breaks down. Alcohol makes the body less aware of cold, depresses heat production through shivering, and can cause a sudden fall in blood sugar (hypoglycemia), especially when taken before exercise, because it depresses the mobilization of glucose from muscle glycogen stores. Alcohol is a serious potential hazard in the outdoors, even though a nip of brandy may do wonders for the spirits of a cold, demoralized person.

BODY HEAT GAIN
Radiation — Sun and fire heat directly by radiation.

Exercise — Voluntary muscle work can produce up to 15 times the normal amount of body heat; involuntary shivering, 6 times. Exhaustion, alcohol and/ or inadequate food or water decreases shivering.

Food — Metabolism of food produces energy that is converted into heat. An average sized adult male requires 4,000 calories each day for heavy work, equivalent to the energy consumed by walking 20km (12 miles) and climbing 750m (2,500ft). Carbohydrate is most quickly absorbed as sugar. Hot food and drink boost morale but transfer meager heat to the stomach. Beware of eating snow to slake thirst; the same amount of heat is needed to melt snow to water as to bring that water to the boil.

Symptoms and signs of hypothermia

MILD HYPOTHERMIA — core temperature 37°C-33°C (98°F-91°F).
The victim can usually still talk; he grumbles and mumbles about
feeling cold, stiff muscles and cramps. Skin is cold, pale and
blue-grey owing to constricted blood vessels and sluggish
circulation. Uncharacteristic behavior is common but may be
obvious only to someone who knows the person's usual personality
and performance. Excitement, lethargy, poor judgement and
decision-making, are common features. Therefore he must never
be left alone, or allowed to wander off.

At a core temperature of about 35°C (95°F) he fumbles and
stumbles because of poor muscular co-ordination. The brain is
fuddled and he may hallucinate and shiver uncontrollably.

Act: the leader must decide whether to escape from the cold,
wind and wet, or to stay put, shelter and summon help, which
may take several hours to arrive.

If the victim appears fit to go on, rest first. Shelter out of the
wind, eat some food and brew a hot drink. Thus boosted he may
be able to descend unaided. But don't sit around too long or he
may cool further, as will his companions. Walk at his pace, not
yours, to a camp or hut where he can be thoroughly warmed.

SEVERE HYPOTHERMIA — core temperature below 32°C (90°F)
Severe hypothermia occurs in wet and cold environments especially
in misadventures on mountains and on water. Shivering stops and
with it disappears the victim's last self-protective mechanism. His
behavior may be irrational and apathetic, or aggressive and
violent. Muscles become stiff and movement is un-coordinated,
breathing slow and pupils are dilated. He may have a seizure and
slip into a coma. An irregular pulse heralds loss of control of the
heart-beat. This all happens fast, and kills. The body core needs
heat urgently during the first half-hour after rescue.

Act: on site
Shelter: the victim out of wind, rain and snow. Erect a tent, dig a
snow-hole, build a lean-to, or put him in a bivouac sack or a
strong polythene bag. Insulate him well from the cold ground with
a closed-cell foam mattress, packsacks or foliage and grass. A fit
companion should climb naked into a sleeping bag beside the

unclothed victim. Inside the sleeping bag place a hot water-bottle, or heated stones wrapped in cloth to prevent burning, or use commercially produced "heat-packs". When the victim is warm dress him in dry clothes and continue to keep him warm.

Rescue: other members of the party may also be cold and miserable and will need sustenance for the long, hard job of rescue. Crowd into a shelter, light a stove and brew a drink — even a single candle will warm a small enclosed space. But beware of poisonous carbon monoxide gas accumulating from stoves.

Leave at least one person to look after the victim. Send the strongest competent member of the party for help, having agreed on a signal to direct arriving rescuers to the victim. Write down the map reference and send it together with a written message about the condition of the victim. Radios and helicopters have greatly simplified modern rescues.

Having decided to stay put and shelter do not waver even if the victim improves; by starting out he may relapse and you may miss the rescuers. Making a hypothermic person walk will further exhaust him. However, if forced to carry him immobile on a stretcher wrap him well because he may continue to cool.

If you have to walk because help is unavailable, plan an escape route that avoids windy places. If the victim is on a stretcher handle him very gently to avoid triggering lethal heart irregularities (arrythmias), and carry him head slightly downhill to maintain his blood pressure. One person should watch him closely all the time. Ideally, start intravenous fluids before the evacuation begins.

Warm, humidified air breathing: re-warming can be started in the wilderness with a portable apparatus that provides heat transfer directly to the core via the big blood vessels of the neck and chest; it also prevents further heat loss from expired air. Such first-aid treatment in the field is a useful adjunct to adequate body insulation.

In one system (U-Vic Heat Treat) air or oxygen passes through a heater-vaporizer unit at 70ºC and into a reservoir re-breathing bag attached to a mask. Another system (Lloyd) generates heat and moisture by passing oxygen through soda-lime previously charged with a pre-set volume of carbon dioxide. The temperature and humidity depend on the volume of carbon dioxide added.

At Base Camp

Hot bath re-warming used to be advocated in the field, but it is now thought that the hypothermic victim should not be actively re-warmed until under total physiological control in hospital. This is fine in theory but in a wilderness hypothermic incident it may be several days before such ideal circumstances obtain. Therefore I suggest the person be allowed to re-warm slowly at his own pace without applying external heat, but in a sleeping bag for comfort. The danger of this period is of re-warming shock due to the sudden return of cold blood to the core carrying with it toxic metabolites of blood pooled in the cold shell.

Re-warming shock — blood pressure falls and pulse rises over 160 per minute and is irregular; it can cause fatal irregularities of the heart (ventricular fibrillation) and CPR may be necessary. Arrythmias are very difficult to diagnose in the field; all are bad news, especially in anyone who is unconscious, under the age of 10 years or over 70, or has a history of heart disease.

Fluid replacement: all hypothermics are short of fluid (dehydration), so give lots of fluid by mouth provided the victim is conscious. Hot bath re-warming shunts blood from core to shell causing more dehydration and shock.

If intravenous fluid is available give 1 to 2 liters of Ringer's lactate or normal saline immediately depending on size. Follow this with 5% dextrose-water (500ml every 6 hours) in order to help transfer glucose across cell membranes and to move potassium back into the cells. Place the i/v bag under his bum so his body weight makes a head of pressure, warms the fluid and prevents it freezing. Give sodium bicarbonate (50 mEq in 50ml = 1 ampule) in the first bag of fluid in order to neutralize the acidity of the blood.

Other re-warming methods are possible only in a well-equipped hospital:

Peritoneal dialysis: flushing warm dialysate fluid round the abdominal peritoneal cavity provides heat directly to the core and helps the body fluid equilibrate with the dialysate.

Extra-corporeal re-warming via cardio-pulmonary by-pass: provides total control and is ideal for the desperately ill, severely hypothermic patient.

IMMERSION HYPOTHERMIA

Immersion hypothermia differs from outdoors exposure in its rapid onset and faster cooling when exercising (e.g. swimming). Water causes heat loss 20 times faster than air because water is an excellent conductor and a large amount of heat is needed to raise its temperature. The victim may drown because hypothermia causes loss of consciousness.

Experiments have shown that volunteers, lightly clothed, floating motionless, immersed to the neck in calm water will reach "incipient death" in 2½ to 3 hours at 10°C (50°F), in 2 hours at 5°C (41°F), and in 1½ hours at 0°C (32°F). Rough seas will shorten these projected survival times, but protective clothing will prolong survival even in rough seas.

A person can swim less than 1km in water at 10°C (50°F) so it will usually be safer to stay with an upturned boat than to strike out for shore. Crouching in a fetal position minimizes heat loss from thermogenic areas of the axilla and groin, and limits burning calories in fruitless attempts to swim in order to keep warm. A personal flotation device (PFD) prolongs survival threefold. Wool insulates better than any other normal clothing when wet. Covering the head reduces heat loss from convection by half. It is warmer out of the water clinging to an upturned boat, despite wind and rain, than staying immersed. Staying with the boat increases the chance of being spotted by searchers. Despair is the overwhelming emotion of a shipwreck victim, who is inclined not to bother with details of survival skills that can tip the balance from death to life.

DEEP HYPOTHERMIA

At temperatures below 28°C (82°F) a person may appear dead; shivering is absent, muscles are stiff like rigor mortis, and skin is pale and bloodless. Heart beat and breathing are barely perceptible. But although oxygen for the brain and heart is greatly diminished, it may be adequate for the body's needs at that temperature.

Declare a victim of hypothermia dead only when warm and dead; that is if he has failed to revive after adequate re-warming. A severely hypothermic victim who is still alive may have fixed and dilated pupils, a common sign of death. The only sure signs of death are no response when the victim is re-warmed, and EKG evidence of the heart having stopped. So do not give up too readily; "corpses" have been known to wake up in a warm mortuary.

18   FROSTBITE

Frostbite is localized freezing injury of tissue of the body shell affecting the face, hands and feet most commonly. Hypothermia, by contrast, is generalized cooling of the deep inner core and contributes to frostbite. If the core remains warm the extremities are less likely to freeze in severe cold weather. Once frostbitten a person seems more susceptible to frostbite again in the same place owing to local nerve damage.

After an accident damaged tissue freezes readily and the chance of frostbite increases because the victim may be immobilized by pain and therefore unable to exercise in order to produce heat. Likewise, shivering may be abolished if the victim is unconscious. Blood loss from an open wound or into a closed fracture causes clinical shock, vessels in the extremities constrict so as to shunt blood from the limbs to the core in order to maintain vital functions. Emotional shock caused by fear resulting from an accident has similar results.

At high altitude the risk of frostbite is great because less oxygen is available to nourish the tissues. Over 6,000m (20,000ft) work is exhausting, sleep is elusive and the brain is dulled, so common sense precautions against cold are often forgotten.

Cold deserves profound respect because frost bites the unwary causing devastating disability. But in the main frostbite is preventable.

Prevention

BODY PROTECTION
A windproof, waterproof suit protects against hypothermia. When insulation is destroyed by wind and water the body core cools and the extremities are in danger of frostbite.

FEET
Tight boots cramp the circulation and cause blisters. Broken skin is liable to cold injury and infection. Stop and remove boots as

soon as the feet feel very cold or begin to lose sensation. Early warming may prevent trouble later. Wear gaiters to keep out snow. Carry spare dry socks, to double as mittens; a wrinkled sock in a boot causes uneven pressure and interferes with blood flow. Windproof trousers keep warm the legs, and hence the feet.

A plastic bag pulled over the foot next to the skin makes a vapor-barrier liner, which traps the warm moisture of sweating feet preventing socks from becoming soaked. At $-40°C$ ($-40°F$) and zero humidity the feet are quite comfortable and, surprisingly, don't feel like standing in a swamp. Rubber vapor-barrier boots are very warm but bulky — good for plodding round camp, but clumsy for technical climbing. Plastic double-skinned climbing boots are warm, waterproof and do not freeze like leather boots do.

HANDS
Outer mittens allow fingers to move freely and to warm each other by contact, whereas gloves isolate each finger. Clothed hands still need to be able to handle equipment like ropes, ice-axes, and crampon straps. In severe cold get in the habit of doing all routine tasks wearing mittens because each time they are removed hands cool quickly. Silk or polypropylene gloves can be worn if mittens have to be removed for performing delicate manual tasks like handling cold metal. Elastic cuffs of jackets and mittens should not be tight. In extreme cold skin sticks to freezing metal so beware of metal spoons and mugs, and never hold metal between the lips.

FACE
The face is difficult to cover completely even with neoprene face-masks; ears and noses cool fast because a large area of skin projects from the face. Carry a pocket signal mirror to inspect frequently cheeks and nose for white patches of frostnip, which appear before any pain is felt. A balaclava wool hat with a visor opening will protect most of the face. A scarf tied loosely over the mouth and nose will ice up with frozen breath forming a barrier to the cold air. Breathing very cold air can cause wheeze like asthma and if prolonged can damage the small terminal air sacs ("frozen lung").

GENITALS

Men have the bigger problem. Fortified under-pants, a rabbit skin
or newspaper stuffed down the front keeps everything warm.
Dipping in brandy does not help.

MECHANISM OF FROSTBITE

Fluid within the cell freezes, the nucleus bursts and the cell dies.
Breakdown products of frozen cells are released on re-warming and
further damage the tissues. Small arteries in the shell constrict in
response to messages from the temperature-regulating center in the
brain. So warm blood flows to the core at the expense of the
extremities, which freeze. Capillaries are damaged by freezing and leak
causing blisters. Cold red blood cells sludge and clot in the small vessels
preventing oxygen reaching the tissues.

   Climbers at high altitude often have to weather out storms in their
tents; they lack exercise to stimulate circulation, and fail to drink
enough because fuel for melting snow is scarce. Red blood cells multiply
in response to oxygen lack, causing blood to become viscous and to flow
sluggishly. Small clots form in the leg veins, pieces break off and lodge
in limbs and lungs.

Symptoms and signs of frostbite

Frostbite behaves like a skin burn and may be superficial or deep
depending on whether there is damage to the germinal layer of the
skin from which new cells arise. Depth of freezing depends on
temperature and length of exposure to cold.

SUPERFICIAL FROSTBITE

Superficial freezing (frostnip) damages only the surface cells, so
complete healing can be expected without loss of tissue. Frozen
tissue is white, waxy, and feels intensely cold, but is soft and
resilient when pressed. The skin tingles and is painful, indicating
that nerves are undamaged. Blisters may form.

   Act: jump up and down to get warm, wriggle toes, flex ankles,
clap hands and swing arms. Put a cold hand in your own armpit
or crotch, or pee on your fingers. Place a cold foot against the
warm trunk of a fit, sympathetic companion. If ears or nose feel
numb hold a warm hand against them or ask a friend to breathe
on them. Never rub snow into a frozen part because snow crystals
act like broken glass. Rubbing the skin vigorously may break the
surface and allow infection to enter. Numbness wears off as the

part thaws giving way to excruciating burning pain.
   Rx: strong analgesics (D.1.3 or 4).

DEEP FROSTBITE

Deep freezing kills tissue and nerves leading to insidious loss of pain and cold sensation. Skin forms blisters and turns a mottled blue. Frozen tissue feels solid to touch; muscle may be frozen, but tendon is usually spared, and frostbitten limbs can still move. The ugly appearance of frostbite, ranging from a patch of black skin, to gangrene of the whole limb, is a poor guide to how much tissue will die eventually — so be not hasty with the knife.

   Act: in the field — rest the frozen limb and keep it clean to prevent infection; dead slough will usually separate from healthy tissue in 2 to 3 months provided there is neither infection nor further damage. Cells at the edge of an area of frostbite are balanced precariously between life and death and need mollycoddling in order to ensure they survive. Don't risk infection by pricking blisters, which if left alone dry over several weeks forming a black crusted scab. Cover the wound with a plain, dry, non-stick dressing. Splint the limb.

   A deeply frozen limb feels tight and is difficult to move; later it swells. Elevate the limb on a rucksack above body level in order to let edema fluid drain away. Once a limb is thawed keep it warm, at rest and protected from further injury. A re-warmed and thawed person should preferably be carried on a stretcher. It is better to walk with feet still frozen before re-warming them because thawing and re-freezing does more damage than walking on frozen feet. Drain blisters with a sterile needle because they will break anyway while walking; then dress them cleanly. In remote regions the victim will have to rest at night and re-warming is inevitable. Just do the best you can.

   Act: in the valley — a frostbitten person may also be suffering from hypothermia. When he reaches a shelter or base camp warm him thoroughly and make him comfortable. Give plenty of fluids. A wee dram of spirits will cheer, but forbid smoking because nicotine constricts by half the caliber of small arteries. Treat pain and anxiety; then thaw the limb.

Thawing: rapid thawing is less damaging to frostbitten tissue than slow re-warming; the limb is frozen for a shorter time and swelling subsides more quickly. Ice formed between cells melts and salts move across the walls upsetting cell chemistry. Stagnant blood starts to re-circulate carrying away poisonous chemicals formed during thawing.

Rapid thawing can only be done at a base camp where adequate fuel and large containers of water are available. Never thaw a limb in front of an open flame as the flesh may cook. Immerse the frozen limb for 20 to 40 minutes in water at about 42°C (105°F); this feels pleasantly warm to the uninjured hand, but using a thermometer is preferable. Hotter water boils tissue. The frozen limb cools the water-bath so stir in more warm water frequently. Do not heat the bath directly because the temperature cannot then be controlled. Continue thawing until the warmed tissue is soft, pliable, and flushed red. Pain may be severe (see below).

Cleaning and dressing: after washing your own hands thoroughly with soap and boiled water clean the frostbitten area daily with a saline solution made with a tablespoon of salt in a liter of boiled water. Gentle dabbing is sufficient; do not scrub the skin surface. Dry fingers or toes and separate them with dry cotton wool.

If possible leave the frozen part open to the air to allow a scab to form. But do not be tempted to pick at the black scab, which protects underlying healing tissue and must be nurtured like a seed bed.

Take scrupulous care to avoid infection which will convert a dry healing scab into soggy, inflamed, wet gangrene that spreads up the limb destroying as it goes. If the wound has to be dressed use a sulpha cream, and change the dressing at least daily. Exercise the part continually to prevent contracture of joints.

Rx: co-trimoxazole (D.2.2) broad spectrum antibiotic, especially if the line between healthy and dead tissue becomes inflamed. Double the dose if it looks red and inflamed, feels tender and throbs.

morphine (D.1.4), or codeine (D.1.3) for pain.

tetanus toxoid — get a booster dose as soon as possible.

Medical sympathectomy: [phenoxybenzamine] 10mg twice daily for 6 days may combat vaso-constriction.

Vaso-dilators [Ronicol, Priscol]. These drugs used to be fashionable but have no place in the field treatment of frostbite. They cause vessels to dilate giving a deceptively pleasant feeling of warmth as blood surges to the skin surface, but they do nothing for the frostbitten part and much heat is lost thereby with further danger of hypothermia.

HOSPITAL
Sympathectomy (surgical): may help if done in the first 24-48 hours after freezing.
Fasciotomy: should be done early to relieve edema causing pressure on small vessels to the hands or in muscle compartments.
Amputation: may be needed eventually but should be delayed until natural separation has taken place. Frostbite in January may mean amputation in July.

Eschew heroic surgery in the field; spreading gangrene is the only indication for emergency amputation. Guess generously at the extent of irreparable damage; notoriously evil-looking limbs can, and do, recover almost completely.

Other types of cold injury

IMMERSION (TRENCH) FOOT
A non-freezing cold injury caused by prolonged exposure of many days, or even weeks, to cold and wet — without freezing. Mild numbness and a feeling of never being warm may progress to freezing cold injury (frostbite).

CHILBLAINS
Repeated exposure of bare skin to wet, wind and cold, causes red, itchy, tender, swollen skin.

19   ACCLIMATIZATION

Acclimatization starts about 1,500m (c5,000ft) and allows humans to live and work in the oxygen-thin atmosphere of high altitude above 2,500m (c8,000ft). The air breathed at sea-level has four parts nitrogen, and one part oxygen. As we climb the 4:1 ratio of these gases does not change, but their density becomes less; fewer molecules are bouncing around in a given volume of air and the pressure exerted by them falls steadily. Thus an ordinary weather barometer can be used as an altimeter because it registers the pressure gases exert on the earth's surface. At the top of Mt. Everest (8,848m, 29,028ft) the atmospheric pressure is less than one third that at sea-level. Eventually the pressure is no longer adequate to drive sufficient nourishing oxygen into the tissues, especially the nerve cells which demand the most; brain cells deprived of oxygen die in less than four minutes.

Life would be unendurable above 3,000m (c10,000ft) without the physiological adjustments of acclimatization, which compensate for the low pressure of oxygen in the air, and high altitude mountaineering would be impossible. Certainly no man could climb to the top of Mt. Everest without oxygen, a feat now achieved several times.

THE INITIAL RAPID PHASE OF ACCLIMATIZATION (from 1,500m, c5,000ft)
Breathing: at sea-level the rate and depth of breathing are controlled by the level of carbon dioxide waste produced by body tissues burning oxygen. Above 3,000m (c10,000ft) carbon dioxide control is over-ridden by the paramount need to get enough oxygen. Low oxygen pressure in the atmosphere, and hence in the lungs and blood (hypoxia) increases the rate and depth of breathing so carbon dioxide levels in the blood fall briskly until a steady state is reached for that individual at that altitude.

Breathing rate increases because hypoxia triggers the carotid chemo-receptor organs in the neck to stimulate the respiratory center in the brain. With deeper breathing carbon dioxide, which dilutes oxygen in the lungs, is removed more rapidly; its concentration in the blood falls, which in turn dampens the activity of the respiratory center. A delicate balance is struck between two opposing forces, low oxygen and low carbon dioxide pressure, which control the rate and depth of breathing.

Increased ventilation of the lungs, especially on exercise, provides more oxygen for absorption by the capillaries. On the other hand, at altitude the accessory breathing muscles (diaphragm, abdomen, intercostals and neck) burn oxygen, so less is available for the hard work of climbing. Low carbon dioxide makes the blood more alkaline and so to compensate, more bicarbonate is excreted by the kidneys.

Cheyne-Stokes periodic breathing: breathing rhythm commonly changes at altitude, particularly at night; it steadily deepens, rises to a crescendo, then falls off and finally ceases completely for several seconds. Then the pattern starts over again. Carbon dioxide in the blood builds to a level where it stimulates the respiratory center. Breathing then restarts, carbon dioxide is blown off, the stimulus lessens and breathing comes to a standstill. With acclimatization this abnormal behavior of the respiratory center settles down to a new level of stimulation by carbon dioxide.

Heart: beats faster and more strongly, thus increasing the flow of blood (cardiac output). The person feels thumping palpitations in the chest and a dull headache throbbing in time with the pulse. Hypoxia stimulates both the carotid chemo-receptors and the sympathetic nervous system making the heart pump more blood to the lungs. Thereby more oxygen is available to the tissues where it is readily released because of the relative difference in pressure between blood and tissue cells. Many capillaries open to carry more blood to the cells. Pressure in the pulmonary artery rises so lung capillaries are better perfused and the surface area for gas exchange is increased.

THE LATE SLOWER PHASE OF ACCLIMATIZATION

Blood and Plasma: soon after arriving at altitude the volume of plasma, the fluid in which blood cells are suspended, falls by 20 to 30%. This is partly because more urine is passed at altitude, partly because of dehydration caused by sweating with heavy exercise, by overbreathing in the cold dry atmosphere, and partly because of a proven shift from the extracellular to the intracellular space. Water losses are hard to replenish above the snow-line because fuel is scarce for melting snow to provide the normal daily requirement of 4 to 5 liters of water, and stoves work less efficiently at altitude.

Hypoxia immediately stimulates bone marrow to produce more red cells in proportion to the severity of oxygen lack. As a result more hemoglobin is produced to carry more oxygen. At high altitude blood can carry up to half as much oxygen again as at sea-level. As red cells increase and plasma diminishes blood becomes more viscous putting a greater strain on the heart. The circulation becomes sluggish, reducing oxygen delivery to the tissues. Red cells clump forming clots and stack together lessening the surface area for oxygen diffusion. The lazy calf muscles of storm-bound climbers fail to compress the leg veins which should normally pump blood efficiently back to the heart.

Tissues: blood is shunted from non-essential to vital tissues (brain, heart, and lungs). Adaptations in the cells assist the release and uptake of oxygen by mitochondria, the power units of cells. Several complex physiological changes lend towards more efficient use of oxygen; new capillary formation, increased muscle myoglobin and the enzyme cytochrome oxidase.

Acclimatization changes have one common purpose: to make optimum use of what little oxygen is available in the thin air on high. But ironically some of these adaptations defeat their own ends, for example, the blunted response of Sherpas to hypoxia.

Acclimatization is quite idiosyncratic; it starts at different altitudes and proceeds at different rates in different people. Some people are never troubled provided they ascend slowly enough, while others for no obvious physical reason never acclimatize properly however long they remain high, even at relatively low altitude. It is not progressive. After about three months at very high altitude, say above 6,000m (c20,000ft), the climber steadily deteriorates. He sleeps and works poorly, and loses appetite and weight. Retreat to the valleys for a long holiday is the solution.

20 ACUTE MOUNTAIN SICKNESS (AMS)

Acute Mountain Sickness (AMS) is caused by diminished oxygen pressure in the atmosphere and hence in the blood (hypoxia), and strikes those who fail to adapt to high altitude, above 2,500m (c8,000ft). Anyone venturing into the high, cold, thin air is wise to study AMS, which can kill the unwary, the bold and the previously healthy. It affects those who ascend too high too fast, and is usually cured by immediate descent.

Mild AMS has vague, ill-defined symptoms but can drift subtly into Severe AMS, which can kill. Hypoxia sets off a chain of events, the fundamental problem being that body water settles in the wrong places; the brain in High Altitude Cerebral Edema (HACE), and/or the lungs in High Altitude Pulmonary Edema (HAPE), or the tissues of the face, hands and feet.

Mild AMS

Many people who climb high are fit on arrival but feel ghastly over the next couple of days, with headache, insomnia, fatigue, breathlessness, poor appetite, nausea and dizziness. These symptoms usually pass off as they adapt to the low partial pressure of oxygen in the air. But some climbers never get used to the altitude, their symptoms become worse and worse, and some die from HACE or HAPE.

PREDICTING AMS
No one can predict who will suffer from AMS whether it will be mild or severe or when it will strike. Climbers who have performed well at altitude will probably do so again each time they go high. Those who have suffered AMS before may suffer again and at a similar altitude. Fitness and training guarantee no protection, the sexes succumb equally and no age is exempt. The young appear more prone, regardless of exercise and rate of ascent. Weight gain during the ascent means water retention, which bodes ill.

PREVENTING AMS

Allow ample time at various levels of ascent to acclimatize. AMS is likely to occur the higher, the faster, the harder, and the longer the climb. Cold and wind, fear and fatigue, dehydration during rapid ascent and strenuous exercise soon after, and upper respiratory infection all predispose to AMS.

Act: *Climb without haste*; above 4,000m, (c13,000ft) gain height slowly and steadily at about 300m/day and take a rest day every 1,000m. Avoid strenuous exertion soon after arriving at altitude. Carry expedition loads high, dump them and descend in order to sleep low. Keep loads light and rest frequently. High mountains should be approached at a leisurely pace both for pleasure and safety. The first Everest climbers always did so on their march through Tibet. They achieved Herculean feats, reaching over 8,500m (28,000ft) in the early 1920s with primitive equipment and clothing, and oxygen apparatus which they rarely used because it was so heavy and clumsy.

Drink sufficient fluid; 4 to 5 liters, about 16 to 20 cups daily, should balance the heavy fluid losses caused by strenuous breathing in cold, dry, thin air, and in order to pee a clear, colorless, copious urine (1 liter daily, about 2 bursting bladder-fulls, is the minimum acceptable). Dark yellow urine is concentrated, usually indicating dehydration; it may however be part of the water retention of AMS. Avoid alcohol; a hangover simulates AMS and may confuse the diagnosis.

Eat a high calorie diet; with plenty of carbohydrate before and during ascent. A good appetite suggests good acclimatizing. Don't take salt or sedatives.

If despite these precautions a climber gets sick and does not improve on rest, **descend** quickly until he starts to feel better. Even 300m will help; 1,000m may be magical.

Beware the climber who acclimatizes poorly and copes less well than expected for the altitude and his previous performance. Macho types who battle ever upward despite worsening distress are those likely to end up buried under a cairn of stones on the glacier.

SYMPTOMS AND SIGNS OF MILD AMS:
These develop 12 to 48 hours after arriving at altitude.

Headache — the victim's head feels tight, as if blown up like a
balloon, and he may feel giddy and light-headed. Headache often
develops during the night so is present on waking, usually at the
base or the posterior part of the head. If headache persists after
exercise and taking two paracetamol the victim must descend. The
severity of headache and its response to treatment, is often a
measure of the severity of AMS, yet some people are found
unconscious in the morning without any warning.

Fatigue — tiredness usually passes off with rest, fluids and food,
all of which restore normal energy.

Appetite loss, nausea and indigestion — a listless, sick, farting
tent-mate is odious; but gas problems improve with
acclimatization.

Sleep disturbance — difficulty in falling asleep, and frequent
waking occur in the first week but may improve in the second. At
great height it may never improve.

Shortness of breath on exertion (dyspnea) — the chest feels
uncomfortable and tight, but quiet easy breathing resumes after
rest. A raspy cough, caused by the cold dry air, is relieved by
inhaling steam from a boiling pot.
    Cheyne-Stokes periodic breathing is particularly noticeable and
worrying at night. Breathing gradually deepens, is often
accompanied by snoring and rises to a peak in 4 to 5 breaths;
then it diminishes and finally ceases completely for several seconds
so you may, wishfully, think the sleeper is dead. This alarming
pattern then starts all over again. It is removed by taking
acetazolamide.

Shortage of fluid (dehydration) — urine output is low for 24 hours
with a story of not drinking enough and perhaps of exposure to
heat and sun. Thirst rages, mucosae and tongue are dry (also
caused by mouth breathing) and the pulse races. Changes in

posture, for example on sitting from lying down, cause the pulse to rise and a feeling of faintness.

Swelling — peripheral edema makes the face puffy with bags under the eyes, rings on the fingers feel tight and the ankles show the imprint of stocking elastic. Swelling is worst in the morning and wears off after rising.

Act: rest, wait and see. Do not give oxygen because it may fool you into thinking the victim is better. If he has not improved within 24 hours consider he has severe AMS, and: **descend.**

Mild AMS may blend unnoticed into severe AMS. HACE or HAPE become manifest depending on whether body water settles in the brain or the lungs or both. The amount of peripheral edema indicates the severity of AMS, so it is better to make a mistake by diagnosing the condition as severe AMS and to descend, than to underestimate mild AMS. The entire drama can unfold within hours and usually does so at night.

Severe AMS

HIGH ALTITUDE CEREBRAL EDEMA (HACE)
HACE usually occurs above 4,000m (c13,000ft); although less common than HAPE 60% of victims will have HAPE as well. It is like an exaggerated form of mild AMS. Symptoms of HACE and HAPE may overlap so it is difficult to tell which is which. But the victim of severe AMS may die quickly so make a confident diagnosis and act decisively.

Headache — severe, constant and throbbing like a bad toothache or migraine. No relief comes from paracetamol (D.1.1), codeine (D.1.3), a night's sleep or massaging the temples.

Inco-ordination (ataxia) — the victim staggers as if drunk, and fumbles fine movements such as handling a camera. To distinguish ataxia from simple tiredness make him perform the following tasks and compare with a normal person as a control:

Toe-to-heel walking: place the heel of one foot against the toes of the other and walk along a 4m straight line drawn in the snow or on the ground. An ataxic person will sway, stagger and fall over when told to turn round and walk back.

Sitting upright without support: a person with ataxia of the trunk will roll over.

Languor — extreme fatigue is not reversed by rest. Pressure on the brain blunts the intellect. The victim won't talk, eat or drink; he lies curled up in a sleeping bag avoiding contact with the outside world; he is apathetic and isolated, yet irritable and confused. If still active he may show poor judgement and thus make bad mountaineering decisions. Sleep is fitful and punctuated by bad dreams. He may hallucinate, hear voices or see non-existent companions, and be incontinent.

N.B. Both ataxia and languor are common to hypothermia (take the rectal temperature), alcohol intoxication (smell the breath) and opiate drug abuse (look for pin-point pupils).

Vomiting — eventually vomiting leads to dehydration which cannot be replenished by drinking. Urine is scanty and dark yellow.

Coma — finally the drowsy victim becomes unrousable, drifts into coma and may die. Convulsions are rare. Cerebral edema victims can remain unconscious for days and yet recover completely.

HIGH ALTITUDE RETINAL HEMORRHAGE (HARH)
One third of all climbers going very high (above 6,000m, c20,000ft) have hemorrhages in the retina at the back of the eye. The diagnosis requires an ophthalmoscope.

The hemorrhages look like red paint splashed on a wall. Usually they cause no symptoms, however, if the sensitive macula area, which interprets fine vision like reading, is involved a blurred or blank patch (scotoma) may be present in the central vision. These retinal hemorrhages heal in a few weeks and usually leave no scars. Similar hemorrhages tend to occur in the brain and may be more harmful.

HIGH ALTITUDE PULMONARY EDEMA (HAPE)
In HAPE the lungs become water-logged hindering the passage of oxygen across the alveolar membranes into the blood so the victim can drown in his own juice.

HAPE is rare below 3,000m (c10,000ft); it begins 36 to 72 hours after arriving at altitude and is cured by DESCENT. Rest and oxygen may help temporarily. It affects children more than adults, men and women equally. It may be related to severe exertion and rate of climb. It worsens at night when oxygen saturation is low owing to the quiet breathing of sleep and to periodic Cheyne-Stokes breathing, which is exaggerated in HAPE. Those who have gone too high for their own good and have suffered HAPE before may suffer again and at a similar altitude.

Symptoms and signs of HAPE

Shortness of breath (dyspnea) — occurs on slight exertion and is even present at rest. Breathing is irregular and fast at more than 25 breaths/min. The victim does not improve with rest, and is hungry for air. The chest feels full and tight, but there is no actual, pain which distinguishes it from heart attack or pneumonia.

Cough and Sputum — early cough is tickling, hacking, and dry — without sputum. Later the sputum is frothy because of air bubbling through edema fluid in the alveoli, and pink and blood-flecked because of capillary blood leaks. By contrast sputum in pneumonia or bronchitis is yellow-green owing to pus in the alveoli, and high fever is present.

Chest Sounds — crackling, moist sounds (crepitations) like rubbing hair between finger and thumb beside the ear, can be heard with a stethoscope or by placing an ear against the back of the victim's bare chest. The noise is due to air bubbling through fluid and can make a clearly audible rattling sound in both lungs, or on one side alone.

Cyanosis — the lips, face and finger-nails look blue at rest because hemoglobin is less saturated with oxygen than normal. A colored tent will obscure cyanosis, which should be observed in natural light.

Pulse — the pulse will be rapid, more than 110 beats per minute.

Act: DESCENT usually cures severe AMS miraculously.

Immediate descent should not be delayed because of night, inconvenience, experimenting with drugs or oxygen, or in expectation of a mountain rescue team or helicopter — unless descending through difficult terrain in the dark is going to cause unwarranted danger to the whole party. The victim, always accompanied and perhaps carried, should descend at least 300m, preferably 1,000m. The greater and faster the descent, the more swiftly will he recover. Even a modest descent can save life. Once down the victim should stay down until he can be examined by a wise physician.

The forms of treatment listed below play for time but should never take preference over evacuating the victim immediately to a lower altitude. He may just want to lie in bed, sniff oxygen and drink tea; but he needs to DESCEND, if necessary by compulsion.

Rest — prop the victim up, so edema fluid sinks to the bottom of his lungs and pools in his legs. Keep him warm and relaxed because cold and anxiety aggravate AMS.

Oxygen — 100% oxygen flowing at 6 liters per minute given via a tight-fitting mask is optimal, but settle for less if the supply is meager. A change in the victim's color from blue to pink shows the effectiveness of oxygen which may relieve headache and help pulmonary edema; but it is merely an adjunct to, not substitute for, descent.

Fluids — drink enough (4 to 5 liters daily minimum) to maintain a copious flow of clear urine (1 liter daily minimum).

Drugs — clearly it is idiotic to plan an ascent so rapid that drugs must be relied on. However acetazolamide and dexamethasone taken in small doses are currently thought to reduce significantly the chance of getting AMS and the severity should it occur.

Rx: acetazolamide (Diamox) (D.6.2) 500mg slow-release capsule once daily, a mild diuretic that does not help acclimatization but diminishes the incidence and severity of AMS, although useless in treatment. It prevents or reduces AMS symptoms in people such as rescuers who have to ascend hurriedly to altitude if taken on the day of arrival at altitude and for 3 days after. It diminishes

Cheyne-Stokes breathing and thereby improves the quality of sleep and maintains oxygenation in the newly arrived at altitude.

dexamethasone (Decadron) (D.4.2) 4mg twice daily starting on the day of ascent and for 3 to 5 days thereafter for preventing AMS; for treating it, 10mg i/v then 4mg every 6 hours. It is a powerful steroid used in neurosurgery to shrink the brain, hence its beneficial effect in AMS and HACE.

furosemide (Lasix) (D.6.1); 40-120mg by mouth, or 40mg i/v slowly, daily — a powerful diuretic, which can lead to collapse from low volume shock if the victim is already dehydrated. Furosemide may clear the lungs of water in HAPE and reverse the suppression of urine brought on by altitude.

morphine (D.1.4) a powerful analgesic which also allays the crippling anxiety of HAPE. Morphine dilates peripheral blood vessels so blood is shifted away from the lungs thereby easing HAPE. It depresses breathing so must be used with caution in HAPE but never used in HACE.

other drugs; digitalis is useless in HAPE as the victim is not in heart failure. Antibiotics are of value only in the presence of chest infection, with fever, pussy spit and crepitations. Spironolactone and antacids are unproven.

Tourniquets and Intermittent Positive Pressure Breathing have no place in the outdoors.

With good sense Acute Mountain Sickness and its sinister offspring, High Altitude Cerebral and Pulmonary Edema, should not happen. But if they do, descend rapidly to a lower altitude in order to prevent their deadly consequences.

21 IMMUNIZATION

N.B. The specialized drugs mentioned in this chapter are mostly found only here and do not necessarily appear in the general drugs section on p.24-27.

Travelers to tropical and sub-tropical countries can be relatively protected by immunization against certain infectious diseases. Inoculation with a small amount of the organism that causes the disease, or a purified derivative of its toxin, produces immune antibodies, which protect against attacking organisms or their toxins.

Some vaccines require several doses spaced apart, therefore an immunization schedule should be planned three months ahead of intended departure. In emergency a crash course can be given in 15 days. Local public health department will have up-to-date information on international immunization requirements.

IMMUNIZATION SCHEDULE

Ideal schedule	week 1	2	3	4	5	6	7	8	9
Diphtheria/tetanus		x							
Typhoid	x				x		X (optional)		
Cholera		x			x			x	
Polio	x								
Yellow Fever				x					
I.S.G.									x

Crash course	days	1	5	12	15
Diphtheria/tetanus		x			
Typhoid		x		x	x
Cholera	x		x	x	
Polio		x			
Yellow Fever	x				
I.S.G.					x

Anyone suffering from immuno-suppression, eczema or severe allergy, pregnant women or those taking steroid medication (cortisone or prednisone) should avoid immunization. If wishing to travel they should obtain a certificate of exemption from their doctor.

Unexplained fever developing in the tropics, or soon after return therefrom, warrants consultation with a doctor, preferably one with access to knowledge about tropical diseases, who can carry out screening.

Immunizations to be considered

TETANUS AND DIPHTHERIA

These diseases are often fatal. Immunization gives complete protection for which a sore, stiff arm and headache that lasts a couple of days, is a small price to pay. Tetanus (lockjaw) still occurs in Britain and North America although it is more common abroad.

All pre-school children should have been immunized so few adults will have escaped primary immunization. Primary active immunization is obtained by 2 intramuscular injections spaced 8 weeks apart. Protection lasts for 10 years then a booster dose is given. After a dirty wound or an animal bite a booster dose is given if there has been no immunization within the last 5 years, or if there is any doubt about a person being up-to-date with their shots.

Act: clean and debride wounds thoroughly because tetanus spores lie dormant in the soil where horse and sheep manure abound. Tetanus should be treated in hospital with human tetanus immune globulin 3 — 10,000 U i/m and penicillin 1,000,000 U every 4 hours or tetracycline 500mg every 6 hours, each for 5 days.

TYPHOID

Two subcutaneous injections of vaccine prepared from killed bacteria are spaced 4 weeks apart. Have a booster dose if traveling to the tropics where typhoid is endemic. The injections may cause local soreness, headache, fever and malaise for a couple of days, during which time avoid alcohol. The vaccine is not fully protective; scrupulous hygiene with water, food and toilet is the only safeguard.

CHOLERA

Immunization is not recommended for tourists because the risk of cholera is low and the vaccine is poorly effective. Some countries demand a single dose for travelers from an infected area, and the international certificate is valid for 6 months only. Check with public health authorities.

POLIOMYELITIS

Immunization is given to most schoolchildren and lasts a lifetime; it consists of 3 doses of live trivalent oral polio vaccine (OPV), or 4 doses of inactivated polio vaccine (IPV), with an IPV booster every 5 years until age 18. If traveling in places with an increased risk of polio, such as living rough where sanitation is poor (polio virus is carried in feces) anyone under 40 should have a single booster dose of IPV (OPV for those under age 18). Protection from polio is painless; the paralysing disease is deadly.

INFECTIOUS HEPATITIS

Immune serum globulin (ISG) 2ml i/m is given for a visit of less than 3 months; 5ml for longer. Protection is good for 4 months, only partial for a further 2 months against hepatitis A; it lasts for 6 months and should be repeated if the danger of infection persists. ISG should be given after other immunizations because it interferes with antibody formation upon which their effectiveness depends.

Hepatitis A virus is carried in feces and is acquired from infected food and water, or by swimming near a sewage outlet. Jaundice is preceded for 3-7 days by vague, unpleasant malaise. Rest is the only treatment.

The new hepatitis B vaccine is recommended for travelers to highly endemic areas like South-east Asia and sub-Saharan Africa, or those likely to come in contact with blood or secretions of potentially infected persons.

TUBERCULOSIS
BCG immunization is given only to high-risk groups such as medical personel who have a negative tuberculin (Mantoux) skin test.

MEASLES
Anyone born after 1956 who has not had measles, or who has not had the vaccine, should receive a single 1ml dose.

YELLOW FEVER
Immunization is advisable before travelling to infected areas (the forests of Central and South America, and East, Central and West Africa); some countries demand vaccination for travelers from these areas The live virus can only be obtained from officially designated centres; an International Certificate is valid 10 days after immunization and lasts for 10 years.

Yellow fever used to be a common killer but is now quite rare. It is carried by mosquitos from mammals, principally monkeys, to man.

SMALLPOX
Vaccination should no longer be given because smallpox has been eradicated world-wide. But several countries still insist on a valid International Certificate showing vaccination within the previous three years.

RABIES
Immunization is only recommended for travelers anticipating

contact with rabies-bearing animals, or those going into an area where rabies is a constant threat (see p.232).

MALARIA

No immunization is possible against malaria which is caused by mosquito-borne parasites, Plasmodium falciparum, P. vivax, P. malariae and P. ovale. Travelers to endemic areas below an altitude of 1,200m should take chloroquine 300mg base (500mg salt) once weekly from 1 week before arrival until 6 weeks after leaving the endemic area.

Chloroquine-resistance has become a serious problem worldwide — details which should be obtained from the consulates of the countries to which a visit is planned, or the local malaria reference centers. Travelers to chloroquine-resistant areas should take pyrimethamine 25mg + sulfadoxine (Fansidar) 500mg once weekly in addition to chloroquine 500mg, but be aware that Fansidar can cause serious (even lethal) skin complications. Mefloquine is the newest prophyllactic drug and may be advised by local public health officers.

Mosquitos tend to bite around dusk but are discouraged by long sleeves, trousers, insect repellent and by mosquito netting over beds. It only takes one bite from an infected mosquito to pass on malaria, so there is risk even on a brief stop-over in a malarial area. The only protection is common sense. Anti-malarial drugs only suppress the parasite; they must be taken regularly in order to maintain an effective blood concentration, and are not 100% effective.

Malaria attacks are heralded by mild fever and sore muscles, followed in several days by chills and high fever. The victim shivers so violently the bed shakes, teeth chatter, skin is blue and cold, the pulse races. An hour later he becomes hot with a temperature up to 41°C (107°F), is flushed, suffers severe headache and may be delirious. Then the temperature falls, he sweats profusely and feels better again. This cycle may be repeated every one, two or three days. The parasite can be demonstrated under the microscope.

Act: cool the victim. Push fluids to maintain a urine output of more than 1 liter/24 hours.

Rx: chloroquine phosphate 600mg base (1g salt) immediately,

then 300mg base (500mg salt) after 6hrs, then 300mg base per day for 2 days. Follow-up with primaquine phosphate is advised to prevent relapses in P. vivax and P. ovale infections only; Rx: 26.3 mg daily for two weeks.

Hygiene

Water and food are the most common sources of disease because of pollution by infected feces and urine of disease carriers e.g. typhoid, shigella, cholera. People in tropical countries are generally less discriminating about where they defecate, partly owing to ignorance, partly to lack of adequate latrines. Food and drinking water become contaminated directly, or by flies. Disease is prevented by drinking pure water only, eating clean food and disposing of sewage efficiently.

WATER
Hillside springs clear of human habitation and animal grazing should be safe for drinking, but stream and river water is probably polluted. Glacial mud and mica, that give alpine rivers their murky appearance, upset the gut.

Outside Europe and North America all water, even in hotels and restaurants, should be considered unsafe to drink unless boiled; kitchens are probably only as clean as are the toilets. If in doubt about drinking water purify it yourself and only drink boiled water, or tea or coffee made with boiling water. Avoid drinking tap water or using it for brushing teeth. Certain towns, such as Kathmandu, have notoriously polluted civil water supplies.

Water Purification — Boiling: briskly for a few seconds kills most organisms; boiling for 10 minutes kills ameba cysts and hepatitis virus, the only way water can be sterilized properly. The color, taste and smell of water is immaterial provided it has been adequately boiled. This may be difficult at high altitude where the boiling point is lower than at sea-level.

Chemical treatment: tincture of iodine 2% (5 drops/liter for clear water, 10 drops for cold or cloudy water, allowed to stand for 30 minutes) kills bacteria, giardia and ameba cysts. Chlorine

(10 drops of 1% solution to 1 liter of water) is the basic ingredient of liquid laundry bleach and some water-purifying tablets; it kills most water-borne bacteria, but not ameba cysts or bacteria embedded in solid particles. When large volumes of water have to be purified, and boiling is not practicable, commercial chlorine or iodine bought across the counter will do. The water must be treated for 15 minutes to 1 hour. A pinch of salt added to each liter improves the taste.

Filtration: removes suspended matter and some bacteria giving the water a deceptively clear appearance. Some filters use an iodine exchange resin and though useful for cleaning large volumes of water, are the least reliable way of making it pure. Filters have to be kept scrupulously clean or they lose their efficacy. Water should be boiled after filtration, not before.

DRINKS
Bottled pop, iced drink cubes and Popsicles are only as safe as the water from which they are made. Unpasturized milk must be boiled; powdered milk is only safe if made up with boiled water and stored in a refrigerator. Wine drunk in moderation is harmless but a surfeit upsets the stomach. Contrary to legend, alcoholic spirits do not sterilize the gut.

ICE CREAM
Germs are harbored in ice-cream, both from the ingredients and from subsequent handling. Well-advertised brands with a reputation at stake, should be reasonably safe.

FOOD
Freshly and thoroughly cooked food is safe because bacteria are killed by heat. Avoid pre-cooked and handled food especially where flies abound. Peel all fruit and vegetables; thorough washing is only second best so beware of salads, tomatoes, lettuces, and watercress because human night-soil is often used as a fertilizer in the tropics. Meat should be thoroughly cooked and eaten immediately because raw or under-done beef and pork harbor tapeworms. Beware of inadequately cleaned prawns and shell-fish, which live on sewage and concentrate the organisms.

Strike a balance between worrying obsessively about what you eat and drink, and commonsense precaution. Some early contact with germs and the accompanying dose of the runs is inevitable; immunity gained may protect against further attacks.

PERSONAL HYGIENE
Many toilets are dirty; squatters have to keep balance by holding onto the walls. Take toilet paper because newsprint is rough and fragile, and glossy magazines are impossible. Wash hands carefully with soap and water immediately afterwards. Keep nails short and clean.

Gut problems

Gastro-enteritis, or food-poisoning, causes diarrhea, which means liquid stools; dysentery is diarrhea with blood. Acute diarrhea may follow an influenzal virus illness, or pigging-out on certain foods.

TRAVELERS' DIARRHEA
This causes more trouble than all other medical hazards encountered abroad. It has as many patent remedies as local names (Gippy Tummy, Delhi Belly, Kathmandu Quickstep, Tokyo Trots, Rangoon Runs, Montezuma's Revenge). The causes may include gluttony, change in climate and an upset in bacteria that are normal and necessary in the bowel. Infection may occur with disease-causing organisms carried in water and food e.g. enterotoxigenic Escherichia coli and shigella, less commonly with salmonella and other bacteria and viruses. Diarrhea developing weeks after return from abroad may be due to the protozoa Giardia lamblia.

Wise doctors recommend hygiene rather than drugs to prevent travelers' diarrhea. Much pleasure in traveling abroad comes from eating local food and drinking wine; it is hardly worth going so far for beer, hamburger and hot-dogs. But be moderate to avoid what could be a very expensive and distressing upset gut.

In exceptional circumstances take doxycycline, a long-acting tetracycline, 100mg daily for 3 weeks from the day before departure; it is expensive and has several unpleasant side-effects such as sunlight sensitivity. It reduces the person's own bacterial flora and may increase the risk of more serious enteric infections such as salmonella.

Travelers' diarrhea is usually an acute, explosive, self-limiting illness that is accompanied by vomiting and feeling groggy because of dehydration from loss of body water; it clears in several days.

Act: go to bed and drink unlimited fluids (at least 500ml an hour of plain boiled water). Eat moderately; dried toast or peeled, grated apple turned brown (pectin) may help to solidify the stools. A short period of starvation in a well-nourished person does no harm, but some travelers living on a shoe-string may be malnourished so further starvation will not help.

Fluid loss: if diarrhea becomes severe with loss of large volumes of water (and accompanying electrolytes) like in cholera, the person may rapidly become dehydrated. Fluid can be replaced according to the WHO formula (D.18) (see p.40).

Sip one glass (250ml) after each bowel movement, or more if still thirsty or if the urine is scanty or yellow and concentrated. If less than 10 watery stools are passed a day drink 1 to 2 liters every 24 hours; if more than 10, sip 1-2 liters every 6 hours. On an expedition abroad carry several packets of ready-measured powder, of which many commercial preparations are available.

Anti-motility drugs: slow the gut's peristaltic contractions, and ease diarrhea and cramping pains, but they may prolong bacterial illness by slowing excretion of bacteria and toxins. Most are related to the narcotic drugs so may cause drowziness. Do not use for more than 2 to 3 days.

Rx: codeine phosphate (D.1.3) 15 to 30mg every 8 hours and loperamide (D.9.3) 4mg every 8 hours can be given together.

Antibiotics should not be used blindly because they kill normal bacteria, which are necessary for gut function, as well as toxin-producing bacteria; also they encourage antibiotic-resistant strains of E. coli to emerge. Antibiotics play little part in speeding recovery and they may prolong the excretion of bacteria during convalescence. The risk of using them prophylactically may outweigh the benefits.

If severe diarrhea (more than 6 stools per day) does not stop after 24 to 48 hours on this treatment, or if blood appears in the stools, go to a hospital for a stool examination.

Rx: co-trimoxazole (D.2.2) 1 to 2 tabs every 12 hours for 3 to 5

days. If diarrhea persists nonetheless presume it may be due to
giardia; Rx: metronidazole (D.2.3) 250mg every 8 hours for a
week.

Others medicines: many popular brands of diarrhea medicine
are at best useless (Kaopectate alters the consistency of the stool
and relieves discomfort for those who have to keep moving), at
worst dangerous (iodohydroxyquin "Entero-vioform" can cause
blindness). Avoid them.

SHIGELLOSIS (bacillary dysentery)
This condition has a sudden severe onset with urgent, explosive
diarrhea that may contain blood, mucus and pus, and causes
griping abdominal cramps. The temperature and pulse rise
quickly. The victim has shivering rigors and feels sick but usually
does not vomit. Shigellosis is similar clinically to amebic dysentery
(see below) and can only be diagnosed accurately by culturing the
offending shigella organism from the stool. Antibiotic sensitivity
can then be tested and the appropriate drug prescribed. Prevent
shigella by taking all the measures described above for travelers'
diarrhea; but do not use anti-motility drugs which can intensify
the illness and delay excretion of toxic organisms.

Rx: co-trimoxazole (D.2.2), amoxycillin or chloramphenicol
250mg every 8 hours is empirical treatment.

CHOLERA
This rare disease is spread by fecally contaminated water and raw
shellfish. Sudden onset of profuse, watery diarrhea with cramps
and collapse due to dehydration (sometimes within a few hours) in
a known epidemic area is cause to suspect cholera. Fluids and
electrolytes must be replaced urgently.

TYPHOID (enteric fever)
Fever increases in spiky fashion over 1 to 3 weeks and may reach
40°C (104°F), accompanied by vague abdominal pain and cough.
Constipation at first may, rarely, turn to bloody, pea-soup
diarrhea. Less common symptoms are headache, a flushed face
and rose-colored spots on the trunk. Eventually the victim
becomes prostrate and desperately ill.

Rx: chloramphenicol, the drug of choice, 500mg every 6 hours for 2 weeks, but it has serious side-effects so should only be administered after reaching a bacteriological diagnosis. Co-trimoxazole (D.2.2) 2 tabs every 6 hours or amoxycillin 2g every 6 hours are second choice. Under medical supervision only, dexamethasone (D.4.1) 4mg every 6 hours for 1 week reduces symptoms and the likelihood of the dangerous complication of perforation of the bowel.

Parasites

AMEBIASIS (Entameba histolytica)
Dysentery may develop gradually over a month but the majority of infected persons are asymptomatic carriers. At the start 3 to 4 loose, foul-smelling stools are passed daily; this increases to a dozen with blood flecks, slimy mucus, painful straining and colicy pain on the right side of the abdomen. Liver abscess is a dreaded late complication but is usually not related to an attack of amebic dysentery.
   Rx: metronidazole (D.2.3) 750mg every 8 hours for 1 week.

GIARDIASIS (Giardia lamblia)
Crampy diarrhea persisting after the return of a traveler is suspicious. Beaver and many other wild and domestic animals carry the parasite and infect surface water supplies. If not treated diarrhea may become chronic with malabsorbtion, weight loss and upper abdominal pain like peptic ulcer or gall-bladder disease.
   Rx: metronidazole (D.2.3) 250mg every 8 hours for 1 week. Avoid alcohol.

WORMS
Worms are a chronic cause of ill-health in the tropics and can be prevented by careful hygiene. Usually one dose of the appropriate drug cleans out the worm, the ova of which must be identified by microscopy of the stool.

Round worm (ascaris), thread or pin worm (enterobius), and whipworm (trichuris) — the worms, or part of them, may be seen in the stool. An itchy bum is sometimes the first warning of enterobius. Worms can mimic appendicitis, which is a rare disease

in natives of the tropics, so surgeons should go easy on the knife.
   Rx: mebendazole 100mg twice daily for 3 days.

Tapeworm (taenia) & diphyllobothrium — thrive in under-cooked
beef, pork and fish. Segments of the worm are passed in the stool
but the head remains attached to the gut and must be killed to
prevent it growing into another worm.
   Rx: niclosamide 2g in 2 doses an hour apart, while fasting.

Hookworm (ankylostoma) & strongyloides — larvae enter through
abrasions on the feet so wear shoes in infected regions. Anemia
may result from heavy and chronic infections.
   Rx: mebendazole 100mg twice daily for 3 days.

Schistosomiasis (bilharzia) — the infective stage of this fluke lives
in fresh water and enters the body through unbroken skin, so
beware of drinking from, or paddling or swimming in, slow-
flowing rivers or lakes. The veins of the bladder or intestine are its
favorite haunt, so blood may be passed in the urine.
   Rx: praziquantel 40mg/kg as a single oral dose.

23   BITES

Wash any bite, including human, with copious water and soap
because mouths are full of bacteria. Any sign of infection —
redness around the wound, or enlarged, tender neighbouring
lymph glands — should be treated with an antibiotic. Check the
victim's tetanus immunization is up-to-date; if not, remind him to
get a booster dose soon.

Animal bites

RABIES
Should be considered after an animal bite, especially in the tropics
or in an endemic area. Although rare, rabies kills. Dogs are the
commonest vectors but foxes, the wolf family, skunks, racoons
and bats can all carry rabies; rabbits, squirrels, chipmunks, rats
and mice never do. Rabies virus lives in the saliva of an infected
animal, whose nervous system becomes affected causing the
frothing of mad dogs; the virus enters humans through a break in
the skin, or possibly by breathing the air in caves inhabited by
rabid bats. Most domestic animals in the western world are
immunized against rabies; not so in the tropics.

Prevention — if bitten or licked by a suspect animal, wash the
wound liberally with soap and water and leave it open to the sun
because ultra-violet light kills some viruses. Cage any suspect
animal; if not possible, shoot it. If the animal is alive and free of
rabies after 10 days, the victim of the bite is safe; if it develops
signs of rabies kill it and send the head, carefully wrapped, to a
laboratory for examination of the brain. If the result is positive for
rabies, or immediately after the bite of a known rabid animal,
start a course of anti-rabies vaccine. Once rabies is manifest with
painful spasms, especially on swallowing (causing hatred of water
— hydrophobia), and excitement leading to convulsions and
paralysis, there is no hope of recovery.
   Rx: rabies immune globulin (RIG) 20 IU/kg in one dose as

soon as possible after exposure + human diploid cell vaccine (HDCV) 1ml i/m at different sites on days 0, 3, 7, 14, 28 & 90.

TULAREMIA

This condition is caused by handling diseased or dead rabbits and beavers. When the organism is inoculated by thorns and briars, ulcers and enlarged lymph glands develop. Seek medical advice.

Snake bites

Less than 1 in 20 persons bitten by snakes die from snake-bite poisoning. North America has pit vipers (rattlesnakes, cotton-mouths, copper-heads), and coral snakes. Viper venom can cause immediate painful stinging inflammation at the bite site, and tissue sloughing. Occasionally a severe body reaction occurs with shock, chills, vomiting and convulsions. Breathing and kidney failure follow. Coral snakes rarely bite but if they do the reaction may be delayed 12 hours, when the victim suddenly collapses. Cobras and legion deadly snakes abound in the tropics, so consult an appropriate book.

When in a snake area wear boots, carry a stick and a flashlight at night, and examine clothes, footwear and sleeping bag before climbing in. Snakes only attack when frightened or provoked. If possible kill the snake without damaging identifying marks around the head; pick up the head cautiously because it can strike up to an hour after being cut off. Take the snake's head and the victim to the local hospital, which may keep anti-venom against the local varieties of poisonous snakes.

Act: wash the bite thoroughly with soap and water. Do not suck or slash the skin over the bite, or pee on it. Bandage firmly and tightly over the bite around the entire limb, splint it, and keep it dependent in order to reduce venom entering the blood stream. Do not freeze or use tourniquets, which can lead to gangrene of the limb. If cobra venom has been spat into the eyes irrigate them thoroughly.

Rx: antivenom 50 to 400ml immediately depending on the severity of the poison. Be sure the victim has actually been bitten because horse serum, from which the anti-venom is made, can cause grave hypersensitivity reactions and anaphylactic shock.

Treat pain and give reassurance because a snake bite strikes terror into the heart. Give a tetanus booster if not up-to-date. Do not use antibiotics unless infection follows.

SCORPIONS, SPIDERS, CATERPILLARS,
CENTIPEDES AND LEGION CREEPY-CRAWLIES
Bites may be venomous causing symptoms varying from local pain to shock and collapse. Dust 10% DDT powder in places like outhouse seats where the beasties may lurk and give a nasty bite.

Rx: similar to snake-bite. Antivenom is available against scorpions and spiders (Black Widow). Local anesthetic injected into the site may ease the pain.

Insect bites

BEES, WASPS, AND HORNETS
Stings can be painful and unpleasant. They can also kill a sensitive or allergic person by anaphylaxis, a reaction which causes giant welts (urticaria), severe wheezing, tight chest, stridorous choking and shock. Allergic people should be skin tested; if they are positive and have had a severe reaction before, they should have venom de-sensitizing injections (which may themselves cause a grave allergic reaction) every 4 weeks indefinitely during the season. They should wear a Medic-Alert medallion and carry a kit containing 2 ampules of adrenalin 0.3ml of 1:1,000 solution in pre-loaded syringes with a needle attached.

Act: remove the sting with tweezers. Apply a hot compress. Neutralize the venom; bee venom is acid so apply bicarbonate of soda or weak ammonia; wasp venom is alkaline so use vinegar or lemon juice. Anti-histamines (D.3) ease the itch.

Rx: adrenalin (D.7.2) 1:1,000, 0.3ml i/v (slowly), s/c, or i/m for severe allergy or anaphylaxis; if in severe shock, repeated every ½ hour. Beware! adrenalin can cause the pulse to race and beat irregularly.

MOSQUITOS AND BLACK FLIES
Mosquitos are described under Malaria (see p.223). Black flies, "no-see-ums", thrive in the sub-arctic. They penetrate mosquito netting and give a vicious bite out of proportion to their tiny size.

Danger comes from infection of the bites because of wild scratching.

SCABIES, LICE, NITS, FLEAS AND BED BUGS
Scabies mites burrow under the skin of the trunk and limbs (everywhere excluding the face) causing intense itching worse at night in a warm bed. Tiny red spots are visible at the bite, and scratch marks are everywhere. Lice (pediculus) lay eggs (nits), which are cemented to the hair of the head and pubis, and in clothing seams. Fleas cause intense itching and leave a trail of bites around the midriff. Bed bugs bite and smell, but do not carry disease.

Rx: malathion for scabies; apply one thin layer of the lotion all over the body excluding the face, leave it for 24 hours, then shower. Repeat once in a week if necessary, or use benzyl benzoate nightly for 3 nights. Hot wash all clothes and bedding, air sleeping bags in the sun, and treat the family or tent-mates likewise. For lice do a single shampoo of one tablespoonful for 4 minutes, then rinse and dry.

LEECHES AND TICKS
Leeches are troublesome in rain forests and tropical marshes. The first sign may be a bootful of blood at the end of the day because bites are painless and prevent blood clotting. Leeches find their way into laced boots, so open sandals have the advantage that you can see them early and deal with them. A flick of a finger, a touch of salt, a lighted cigarette or tincture of iodine makes the leech drop off; do not pull them or the head will be left in the wound and continue to irritate. Clean the wound with soap and water, and press to stop bleeding.

JELLYFISH, STINGRAYS, SEA ANEMONES
Stings from these sea creatures cause intense burning pain, local swelling and red wheals. Sometimes the victim is prostrated.

Rx: as for other bites.

ITCHING
Itching can drive a person crazy, literally; more scratch, more itch. Dirty finger nails will turn a bite septic.

Rx: calamine lotion soothes and cools more than cream; starch or oatmeal paste is made by adding 1 cup to 1 liter of boiling water and applying the paste when cool to the area.

anti-histamines quell itching (promethazine (D.3.1) but cause drowsiness (chlorpheniramine (D.3.2) is the least soporific). Anti-histamine creams can sensitize the skin to oral anti-histamines taken later and a violent skin reaction may result. Only use betamethasone (D.11.1) steroid cream if other methods fail.

INSECT REPELLENTS
Applied to the skin they repel insects for 4 hours maximum.

Rx: an insect repellent containing DET (diethyltoluamide), or DMP (dimethylphthalate)

INSECTICIDES
The clothing and the person wearing it must be treated; crystals of powder or droplets of spray stick to the insect and slowly paralyse it.

Rx: an insecticide containing DDT(dicophane)

ALLERGY
A sensitivity reaction to foreign protein may manifest simply as local swelling with welts and occasionally some wheezing.

Rx: anti-histamine (D.3).

SEXUALLY TRANSMITTED DISEASES
Unfortunately the aphorism "once bitten twice shy" does not always apply to foreign travelers for whom the excitement and availability of commercial sex away from home may cause them to abandon discretion. Some nasty strains of penicillin-resistant gonococci (which cause gonorrhea), treponema (which cause syphylis), and herpes virus exist abroad. AIDS (auto-immune deficiency syndrome) can no longer be considered a unisexual disease and 50% of people, male and female, in some African countries have the HIV antibody. AIDS is also acquired from unsterile injections (particularly in intravenous drug users) and blood transfusions.

Act: don't; it's safer that way. But if caught with your pants down and if a pussy urethral discharge and painful peeing come on following an unwise sexual contact, get to a VD specialist clinic quick.

Rx amoxycillin 500mg every 8 hours for 10 days, or cephalosporin (D.2.1).

Index